Handbook of
Pharmacy
Management

Standard Operating Procedures

Handbook of
Pharmacy
Management

Standard Operating Procedures

Sangeeta Sharma MD, MBA

Professor and Head
Department of Neuropsychopharmacology
Institute of Human Behaviour and Allied Sciences (IHBAS)
and
President, Delhi Society for Promotion of Rational use of Drugs (DSPRUD)
Delhi

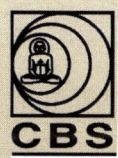

CBS Publishers & Distributors Pvt Ltd

New Delhi • Bengaluru • Chennai • Kochi • Kolkata • Mumbai
Hyderabad • Jharkhand • Nagpur • Patna • Pune • Uttarakhand

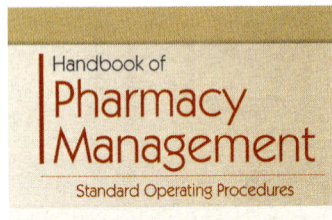

Handbook of
**Pharmacy
Management**
Standard Operating Procedures

ISBN: 978-93-89396-24-9

First Edition: 2021

Published by Satish Kumar Jain and produced by Varun Jain for

CBS Publishers & Distributors Pvt Ltd

4819/XI Prahlad Street, 24 Ansari Road, Daryaganj, New Delhi 110 002, India
Ph: 011-23289259, 23266861, 23266867   Fax: 011-23243014
Website: www.cbspd.com   e-mail: delhi@cbspd.com; cbspubs@airtelmail.in

Corporate Office: 204 FIE, Industrial Area, Patparganj, Delhi 110 092, India
Ph: 011-49344934   Fax: 011-49344935   e-mail: publishing@cbspd.com; publicity@cbspd.com

Branches

- **Bengaluru:** Seema House 2975, 17th Cross, K.R. Road, Banasankari 2nd Stage, Bengaluru 560 070, Karnataka, India
  Ph: +91-80-26771678/79   Fax: +91-80-26771680   e-mail: bangalore@cbspd.com
- **Chennai:** 7, Subbaraya Street, Shenoy Nagar, Chennai 600 030, Tamil Nadu, India
  Ph: +91-44-26680620, 26681266   Fax: +91-44-42032115   e-mail: chennai@cbspd.com
- **Kochi:** 42/1325, 1326, Power House Road, Opposite KSEB, Power House, Ernakulum-682018, Kochi, Kerala, India
  Ph: +91-484-4059061-67   Fax: +91-484-4059065   e-mail: kochi@cbspd.com
- **Kolkata:** 6/B, Ground Floor, Rameswar Shaw Road, Kolkata-700 014 (West Bengal), India
  Ph: +91-33-22891126, 22891127, 22891128   e-mail: kolkata@cbspd.com
- **Mumbai:** 83-C, Dr E Moses Road, Worli, Mumbai-400018, Maharashtra, India
  Ph: +91-22-24902340/41   Fax: +91-22-24902342   e-mail: mumbai@cbspd.com

Representatives

• **Hyderabad**	0-9885175004	• **Jharkhand**	0-9811541605	• **Nagpur**	0-9421945513
• **Patna**	0-9334159340	• **Pune**	0-9623451994	• **Uttarakhand**	0-9716462459

Printed at Goyal Offset Works (P) Limited

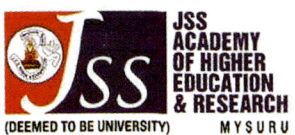
Dr. B. Suresh
Pro-Chancellor

MESSAGE

Over the last several years, the healthcare environment has seen a great deal of change so as the pharmacy practice. In a rapidly evolving health care system with increased demands for results and personalized care, role of a pharmacist has become critical in the provision of care. Historically, pharmacists' role in healthcare was centred on dispensing medications largely. However, over the years, the role of pharmacists has evolved along with the health care needs of the population. In fact pharmacists are one of the key stakeholders of medication management process and contribute in providing medication safety in several ways. With an increasingly wide range of new medicines, medical products, vaccines, and technologies, the complexity of pharmacy practice continues to broaden. Therefore, today's pharmacists need to be competent, up-to-date and possess both vision and a voice to fully integrate principles of patient safety into practice as a member of the healthcare team.

This manual describes on all aspects of pharmacy management and contains step- wise standard operating procedures and clear illustrations on various issues threatening safety in dispensing procedures, adverse event reporting, handling of high alert & lookalike sound alike medicines, medicines requiring special storage conditions (narcotics, thermo-labile products, hazardous medicines) besides fundamental principles of good store management, inventory management, procurement practices etc. On perusal of the content I found a section on quality tools in pharmacy which is very informative and explained jargon used in quality improvement activities in simple language and I hope it will enable pharmacists to actively undertake quality and performance improvement projects and assume a greater role as member of healthcare team in improving quality of pharmacy services.

Pharmacy Council of India has defined the roles and requirements for pharmacy practice under the Pharmacy Practice Regulation Act and continuing pharmacy education for licence renewal. This handbook will be an invaluable comprehensive resource for pharmacists and hope that practicing pharmacists will find it useful in their day-to-day practice.

I congratulate and wish all the best to the author of the handbook.

Dr. B Suresh
Pro Chancellor
& President, Pharmacy Council of India

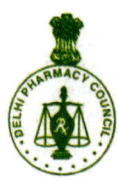

DELHI PHARMACY COUNCIL

(Constituted Under The Pharmacy act 1948)

NATIONAL CAPITAL TERRITORY OF DELHI

Room No. 198, Main Building, Old Secretariat, Delhi-110054
Tel. : 23890034, 23890385 Fax : 011-23890265
Website : www. pharmacy.delhigovt.nic.in
E.mail : slanasa@yahoo.co.in

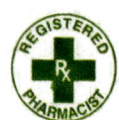

MESSAGE

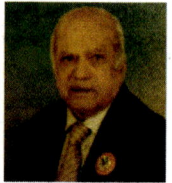

Providing high-quality, safe medical care is the primary goal of health systems. Ensuring safety in the health system is a team effort with pharmacists playing an integral role in preventing and managing medication errors. Role of a pharmacist is critical in the rapidly evolving health care system with increased demands for improved outcomes and patient safety. Drugs and medical supplies are dispensed at the cutting edge level of the interface between the health system and people. Excess drugs or stock outs not only lead to wastage of scarce resources but also bring discredit to a health system. Pharmacists have crucial roles to play in medication management processes right from procurement of efficacious & good quality products, to their dispensing, storage and use. Pharmacists are well positioned to assist the healthcare system in improving quality of care. Pharmacists can help by preventing patients from being harmed by medication. Further, the roles of pharmacists are not only limited to medical products, but also include vaccines and medical devices, especially those that demand special knowledge with regard to uses and risks. Pharmacists ensure the provision of cost-effective health care through rational use of medical products and modern technologies.

Well-performing pharmacists are responsive to patient's needs and preferences. Pharmacists are experts in field of medicine management and provide a range of services ranging from selection, purchasing, storage, dispensing, quality, testing & supply, storage, inventory control, security of stores, designing of medical stores/warehouses, transport etc. Each of these areas of pharmacy management is discussed in detail in this manual.

Besides covering all the essential information required to develop competency to provide pharmaceutical care, this handbook addresses important aspects such as safety in dispensing procedure, dispensing to special population, handling of high alert, look alike and sound alike medicines, narcotics, vaccines and hazardous materials. This handbook not only provides good practice requirements but also provides clear answers for those working in resource limited settings. Section on quality tools in pharmacy is a much needed section for pharmacists and will expand their knowledge and broaden their participation in quality and performance improvement projects beyond traditional medication monitoring.

I congratulate the author of this book for developing this handbook and hope that easy-to-understand language with illustrations will equip the pharmacists about prevention of medication errors and all aspects of medicine management.

(SL Nasa)
Registrar, Delhi Pharmacy Council
President, Indian Hospital Pharmacist's Association (IHPA)

Preface

Pharmacists are a vital part of the healthcare team. The role of the pharmacist is to change alongside the changing needs and expectations of the service users i.e., patients. Pharmacy Practice Rules notified in 2015 by Government of India aimed at enhancing the status and practice of pharmacy profession in the country. These regulations are the first comprehensive changes introduced to the outdated provisions in the laws governing the pharmacy practice. The pharmacy practice was earlier regulated by the Pharmacy Act and Drugs & Cosmetics Act, 1940. The new set of Regulations of 2015 lay down a uniform 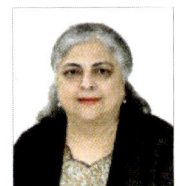 code of pharmacy ethics, responsibilities of pharmacist towards patient, job requirements of a pharmacist, role of a community pharmacist and drug information pharmacist, etc.

Hospital pharmacists are experts in field of medicines, and provide a range of services which can be technical-purchasing, storage, dispensing, quality, testing & supply of all the medicines used in hospitals; clinical pharmacist is an integral part of the healthcare team where the focus is firmly on patient. Drugs and medical supplies are dispensed at the cutting edge level of the interface between the health system and the people. Availability or lack of availability brings both credit and discredit to a health system. On the other hand medicines are double-edged weapons also. If used appropriately, they cure patients but inappropriate use or errors can cause harm to the patients. Several tragedies have occurred due to errors and adverse effects compromising with the patient's safety. Pharmacists have crucial roles to play right from procurement of efficacious & good quality products, to their dispensing, storage and use. Pharmacists can help by preventing patients from being harmed by medication.

In the above context, the proper management of drug supply and good dispensing practices assume paramount importance in the dispensation of health care. In practice it is seen that pharmacists spends more time in non-value tasks leading to waste and errors and often looking for guidance from their peers or learn by making mistakes. The content of the book have been developed to equip pharmacists for the roles they have to undertake in practice and be in line with the standards for pharmacy management. So that pharmacist's can fulfill their major responsibility by spending more time on tasks which add value, such as education, counselling of patients on how to take medicines and medication safety.

This manual describes the good practices in the various processes involved in the pharmaceutical products supply management. Care has been taken to present solutions to issues/problems faced in different settings, during day-to-day practice in a comprehensive manner which otherwise are not available readily. My long years of experience of working closely with the pharmacists and first hand experience of ground realities inspired me to write this book. The guidance is also provided on handling of high-alert, narcotics, hazardous drugs, thermolabile products, vaccines etc. to improve patient safety. The pharmacists can also benefit significantly from applying quality tools and techniques to their pharmacy and key indicators which can be used for monitoring performance. It is intended for use not only by pharmacists (hospital and community setting) who already practice in patient care settings, but also by educators and new students – the pharmacists of tomorrow.

Sangeeta Sharma

Acknowledgements

I would like to express my deep gratitude to Late Professor Ranjit Roy Chaudhury, Late Professor Usha Gupta, both founders of the Delhi Society for Promotion of Rational Use of Drugs (DSPRUD) and Dr. Hans Hogerzeil, then Director, EDM, WHO, Geneva for their able guidance and encouragement to pursue work in this area.

The author wishes to convey grateful thanks to Dr. Govind Miglani for his contributions, Dr. Amit Arya, Dr. Ankit Bhardhwaj, Senior Resident, IHBAS for the suggestions and Mr. Brijesh Gandharv and Ms. Vineeta Bablani, IHBAS for the art work.

I must acknowledge the patience and understanding given by my family especially my husband Mr. Anil Kumar Sharma for the many hours spent by me in writing this book.

Contents

1 | Introduction

Medicines are backbone of therapeutic armamentarium but they are double-edged weapons also. If used appropriately, they cure patients but inappropriate use can cause harm to the patients. Its use has grown dramatically because of increase in life expectancy, increase in the prevalence of chronic disease, emergence of new infectious diseases. Also availability of range of effective medications has broadened because of medicines being used for more and more so-called "life-style medicines" such as baldness, dry skin, wrinkles, erectile dysfunction, etc.

The goal of the healthcare management is to ensure that pharmaceutical services are the best to meet the health care needs of the people. Medication safety has become a major concern all over the world. There are increasing reports of medication errors as one of the leading causes of death and injury due to their misuse and adverse effects compromising with the patient's safety. Medicines have been withdrawn from the market due to unacceptable adverse effects and safety reasons. Nevertheless, medicines moving in the market are not completely safe. It is important for all stakeholders (doctors, nurses, pharmacists and community) to understand medicines properly and use them rationally.

I. NEW DIMENSIONS OF PHARMACY PRACTICE

Pharmacists are one of the key stakeholders of medication management process and contribute in providing medication safety in several ways. The role of the pharmacist has evolved from that of a compounder and supplier of medicines towards that of a provider of patient care and medicines information and education of patients to enhance adherence to the prescribed therapy. Pharmacists help resolve patient questions and can counsel the patients on medication use. They can make a unique contribution to the outcome of drug therapy and to their patients' quality of life by ensuring that a drug therapy is appropriately indicated, the most effective, the safest possible, and convenient for the patient is available.

Access to medicines of assured quality and affordability remains a major concern worldwide. One third of the world's population do not yet have regular access to essential medicines and 50%–90% of medicines purchased are paid for out-of-pocket. This out-of-pocket burden falls most heavily on the poor, who are not adequately protected either by current health policies or by any health insurance. Pharmacists need to ensure that people can access medicines or pharmaceutical advice easily and, as far as possible, in a way and at a time, place of their own choosing and at affordable cost.

In patient-centred health care, the first challenge is to identify and meet the changing needs of patients. Another major challenge is ensuring that medicines are used rationally. *Rational use of medicines requires that patients receive medications appropriate to their needs, in doses that meet their own individual requirements for an adequate period of time, and at the lowest cost to them and their community.* However, rational use of medicines remains the exception rather than the rule.

For those who do receive medicines about 50% medications are prescribed incorrectly and 50% patients fail to take medicines as prescribed. Self-treatment of common ailments is becoming more popular due to over-the-counter easy availability of medicines without the need for a doctor's prescription. Antibiotic misuse, over-the-counter dispensing without prescription and growing antibiotic resistance have become a major public health problem. Pharmacists assume greater role in this setting and provide advise both on the choice of medicines and their safe and effective use. The right choice of self-treatment can prevent some conditions from developing or help others clear up more quickly.

They can empower patients to manage their own health and treatment by offering unbiased relevant evidence-based information. Counselling on how to take medication properly not only improves adherence to medical treatment but also helps in disease prevention and lifestyle modification promoting public health, thus optimizing health outcomes, reduce the number of medicine-related adverse events, cut inappropriate spending on medicines.

Medication management process is vulnerable to a number of 'medication misadventure or error' ranging from inappropriate selection, storage, dispensing, administration of drugs, lack of patient information and prescriber's information.[1] The medication errors cause iatrogenic injury and prolong hospital stay with additional economic burden. Drug complications were the most common type of outcome attributed to negligence, accounting for 19% of these preventable adverse events[2].

Pharmacists can help by preventing patients from being harmed by medication. The number of medicines available in market has increased dramatically over the last few decades, bringing some real innovations but also considerable challenges in controlling the quality and rational use of medicines particularly of the irrational fixed dose combinations. Dispensing errors can be reduced by appropriately managing Look-alike and Sound-alike (LASA) drugs, high alert and high risk drugs. These categories of drugs are one of the major causes for medication errors. Pharmacists can minimize the possibility of drug-drug interactions and allergic reactions and make sure that the patient gets the most benefit from medications.

In hospitals, pharmacists have crucial roles to play right from procurement of efficacious & good quality products, to their dispensing and use. The logistical aspect of distribution – often seen as the pharmacist's traditional role, especially in health institutions – represents another challenge. They can ensure least stock-outs by efficient inventory management.

The quality of medicines can be adversely affected by poor storage and distribution. Although reliable data is not available but it is estimated that in many developing countries 10%–20% of sampled medicines fail quality control tests. Thus maintaining proper storage conditions for health commodities is vital to ensuring their quality. Product expiration dates are based on ideal storage conditions and protecting product quality until expiration date is important for serving customers and conserving resources.

All pharmacists are obliged to ensure that the service they provide is of high quality. The education and training of the pharmacists must equip them for the roles they have to undertake in practice. This hand book on Standard Operating Procedures on good dispensing practices and stock management provides an opportunity to the

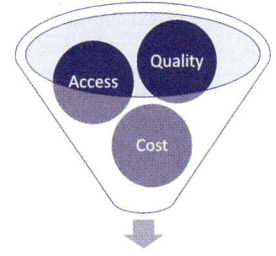

(Often) competing goals

1   Sheldon T. Dutch study shows that 40% of adverse incidents in hospital are avoidable. BMJ. 2007;334(7600):925.
2   Scott M Mark, Jeffery D Little, Sarah Gellar and Robert J Weber. Pharmacotherapy. A Pathophysiologic Approach, 8E, "Principles and Practices of Medication Safety: Introduction."

pharmacists working in the hospitals and community pharmacy to learn and get acquainted with medication safety issues and store management. However, at all stages, the development and improvement of communication skills also needs to be emphasized.

Pharmacists will need to be competent and possess both vision and a voice to fully integrate them into the healthcare team. To do so, pharmacists must assume greater responsibility than they currently do for the management of drug therapies for the patients. They serve and provide guidance on best practices in each of these areas/functions. This handbook describes practical reference for those managing or involved in setting up store-room or warehouse as well. This handbook contains written directions and clear illustrations on receiving and arranging commodities; special storage conditions; tracking commodities; maintaining the quality of the products; constructing and designing a medical store; waste management; and resources. The guidelines and information it contains apply to any storage facility, of any size, in any type of environment.

A. THE UNDERLYING PHILOSOPHY AND THE SCOPE OF PHARMACY PRACTICE

Pharmacy as a dynamic, information-driven, patient-oriented profession, through its infrastructure, competence and skills, is committed to fulfill the healthcare needs of its people by being the:

1. Custodian of medicine;
2. Formulator, manufacturer, distributor and controller of safe, effective and quality medicine;
3. Adviser on the safe, rational and appropriate use of medicine;
4. Provider of accessible, essential clinical services including screening and referral services;
5. Accessible provider of health care information;
6. Provider of pharmaceutical care by taking responsibility for the therapeutic outcome of therapy and by being actively involved in the design, implementation and monitoring of an effective pharmaceutical service;
7. Profession committed to competency and professionalism;
8. Profession committed to co-operation with members of the healthcare team in the interest of the patient; and Profession committed to cost-effective pharmaceutical services.

Over the past 40 years, the pharmacist's role has changed from that of compounder and dispenser to one of "drug therapy manager". This involves responsibilities to ensure that wherever medicines are provided and used, quality products are selected, procured, stored, distributed, dispensed and administered so that they contribute to the health of patients, and not to their harm. The scope of pharmacy practice now includes patient-centred care with all the cognitive functions of counselling, providing drug information and monitoring drug therapy, as well as technical aspects of pharmaceutical services, including medicines supply management.

Pharmacists practice in a wide variety of settings. These include community pharmacy (in retail and other health care settings), hospital pharmacy (in all types of hospital from small local hospitals to large teaching hospitals), the pharmaceutical industry and academia. In addition, pharmacists are involved in health service administration, in research, in international health and in non-governmental organizations (NGOs).

B. THE PHARMACIST AS A MEMBER OF THE HEALTHCARE TEAM

Pharmacists are in an excellent position to meet the need for professionals to assure the safe and effective use of medicines. Pharmacists have the potential to improve therapeutic outcomes and patients' quality of life within available resources, and must position themselves appropriately within the health care system.

The pharmacist's involvement with pharmaceuticals can be in, formulation, manufacturing, quality assurance, licensing, marketing, distribution, storage, supply, information management, dispensing, monitoring or education or research and development. Supply and information management activities have been termed "pharmaceutical services" and continue to form the foundation of pharmacy practice.

THE SEVEN-STAR PHARMACIST

To be effective healthcare team members, pharmacists need skills and attitudes enabling them to assume many different functions. The concept of the seven-star pharmacist was introduced by WHO and International Pharmaceutical Federation (FIP) to describe these roles. The roles of the pharmacist are described below and include the following functions:

1. **Caregiver**: Pharmacists provide caring services. They must view their practice as integrated and continuous with those of the health care system and other health professionals. Services must be of the highest quality.

2. **Decision-maker**: The appropriate, efficacious, safe and cost-effective use of resources (e.g., personnel, medicines, chemicals, equipment, procedures, practices) should be the foundation of the pharmacist's work. At the local and national levels, pharmacists play a role in setting medicines policy. Achieving this goal requires the ability to evaluate, synthesize data and information and decide upon the most appropriate course of action.

3. **Communicator**: The pharmacist is in an ideal position to provide a link between prescriber and patient, and to communicate information on health and medicines to the public. He or she must be knowledgeable and confident while interacting with other health professionals and the public. Communication involves verbal, non-verbal, listening and writing skills.

4. **Manager**: Pharmacists must be able to manage resources (human, physical and financial) and information effectively; they must also be comfortable being managed by others, whether by an employer or the manager/leader of a health care team. More and more, information and its related technology will provide challenges as pharmacists assume greater responsibility for sharing information about medicines and related products and ensuring their quality.

5. **Lifelong-learner**: It is impossible to acquire all the knowledge and experience needed to pursue a lifelong career as a pharmacist in pharmacy school. Pharmacists should learn how to keep their knowledge and skills up-to-date throughout the pharmacist's career.

6. **Teacher**: The pharmacist has a responsibility to assist with the education and training of future generations of pharmacists and the public. Participating as a teacher not only imparts knowledge to others, it offers an opportunity for the practitioner to gain new knowledge and to fine-tune existing skills.

7. **Leader**: In multidisciplinary caring situations or in areas where other healthcare providers are in short supply or non-existent the pharmacist is obligated to assume a leadership position in the overall welfare of the patient and the community. Leadership involves compassion and empathy as well as vision and the ability to make decisions, communicate, and manage effectively.

And the added function of:

8. **Researcher**: The pharmacist must be able to use the evidence base (e.g., scientific, pharmacy practice, health system) effectively in order to advice on the rational use of medicines in the health care team. By sharing and documenting experiences, the pharmacist can also contribute to the evidence base with the goal of optimizing patient care and outcomes. As a researcher,

the pharmacist is able to increase the accessibility of unbiased health and medicines-related information to the public and other health care professionals.

Pharmacists' services and involvement in patient-centred care have been associated with improved health and economic outcomes, a reduction in medicine-related adverse events, improved quality of life, and reduced morbidity and mortality.

C. CLINICAL PHARMACY

The term "clinical pharmacy" was coined to describe the work of pharmacists whose primary job is to interact with the healthcare team, interview and assess patients, make specific therapeutic recommendations, monitor patient responses to drug therapy and provide medicines information. Clinical pharmacists work primarily in hospitals and acute care settings and provide patient-oriented rather than product-oriented services. The medical record, also known as the patient chart or file, is a legal document including hospital-specific admission information, initial patient history and physical examination, daily progress notes made by health care professionals who interact with the patient, consultations, nursing notes, laboratory results, diagnostic procedures, dietary recommendations, radiology and surgery reports. Most charts also include sections for medication orders and clinical pharmacist review progress notes, comments on pharmacokinetic dosing and other relevant therapeutic comments.

Clinical pharmacy requires an expert knowledge of therapeutics, a good understanding of disease processes and knowledge of pharmaceutical products. In addition, clinical pharmacy requires strong communication skills with solid knowledge of the medical terminology, drug monitoring skills, provision of medicines information, therapeutic planning skills and the ability to assess and interpret physical and laboratory findings.

Pharmacokinetic dosing and monitoring is a special skill and service provided by clinical pharmacists. Clinical pharmacists are often active members of the medical team and accompany ward rounds to contribute to bedside therapeutic discussions.

D. PHARMACOVIGILANCE

Medicines safety is another important issue. Because of intense competition among pharmaceutical manufacturers, products may be registered and marketed in many countries simultaneously. As a result, adverse effects may not always be readily identified if are not monitored systematically. Pharmacovigilance is a structured process for the monitoring and detection of adverse drug reactions (ADRs) in a given context.

Pharmacovigilance is defined as the science and activities concerned with the detection, assessment, understanding and prevention of adverse reactions to medicines (i.e. adverse drug reactions or ADRs). The ultimate goal of this activity is to improve the safe and rational use of medicines, thereby improving patient care and public health. Pharmacovigilance includes the dissemination of such information. In some cases, medicines may need to be recalled and withdrawn from a market, a process that entails concerted action by all those involved at any point in the medicines supply chain.

Data derived from sources such as Medicines Information, Toxicology and Pharmacovigilance Centres have great relevance and educational value in the management of the safety of medicines. Medicine-related problems, once detected, need to be assessed, analysed, followed up and communicated to regulatory authorities, health professionals and the public.

Pharmacists have an important contribution to make to post-marketing surveillance and pharmacoviglance. Adverse drug reaction reporting is discussed in detail in the section on Adverse Drug Reaction & Reporting.

II. GOOD PHARMACY PRACTICE REQUIREMENTS

1. A pharmacist's first concern must be the welfare of the patient and of the public in general.

2. The core of pharmacy activity is the supply and distribution of medicines and other health care products, the provision of appropriate information and advice to the patient, ensuring the correct use of medicine and monitoring the effects of the use of medicines (pharmaceutical care).

3. An integral part of the pharmacist's contribution to health care is the promotion of rational and economic pharmcotherapy and optimal use of medicines.

4. The objective of each element of the care provided by pharmacist is clearly defined, relevant to the individual and effectively communicated to and accepted by all those involved.

   i. The ongoing relationship with other health professionals should be seen as a therapeutic alliance involving mutual trust and confidence in all matters relating to pharmaco-therapeutics;

   ii. The relationship with others should be as colleagues, each seeking to improve pharmaceutical services, rather than as competitors;

   iii. There must be input by the pharmacist to decisions on medicine use policy at all levels;

   iv. The relationship with those involved in paying for pharmaceutical services should also be one of mutual trust, involving appropriate professional discretion;

   v. The pharmacist should be aware of essential medical and pharmaceutical information about each person to whom a pharmaceutical service is provided. Obtaining such information is simplified, if the patient chooses to use only one pharmacy; the pharmacist needs independent, comprehensive, objective and current information about therapeutics and medicines in use;

   vi. The philosophy underlying practice should be professionally rather than commercially oriented;

   vii. Store in-charge/pharmacists in each field of practice should accept personal responsibility for the self-assessment and maintenance of competence throughout their professional working lives.

A. THE PHARMACY PRACTICE ACTIVITY CLASSIFICATION

1. Ensuring appropriate therapy and outcomes
   i. Ensuring appropriate pharmacotherapy
   ii. Ensuring patient's understanding/adherence to his or her treatment plan
   iii. Monitoring and reporting outcomes

2. Dispensing medications and devices
   i. Processing the prescription or medicine order
   ii. Preparing the pharmaceutical product
   iii. Delivering the medication or device

3. Health promotion and disease prevention
   i. Delivering clinical preventive services

ii.　Surveillance and reporting of public health issues

iii.　Promoting safe medication use in society

4.　Health systems management

i.　Managing the practice

ii.　Managing medications throughout the health system

iii.　Managing the use of medications within the health system

iv.　Participating in research activities

v.　Engaging in interdisciplinary collaboration

B. QUALITY ASSURANCE OF PHARMACY SERVICES

A basic concept which should underlie all healthcare services and pharmacy practice is that of assuring the quality of patient care activities. Avedis Donabedian, the father of quality assurance, defined the three elements of quality assurance in healthcare as being structure, process and outcome. **Structure** describes the context in which care is delivered or facilities being provided which includes hospital buildings, staff and ratio of staff to patients, waiting time, financing, and equipment. **Process** denotes the transactions between patients and providers throughout the delivery of healthcare. In other words, it includes whether or not good medical practices are followed. Examples include services offered, patient-provider interactions, access, safety, counseling quality, the percentage of people receiving preventive services (such as immunizations or mammograms); the percentage of people with diabetes who had their blood sugar tested and controlled.

Finally, **outcomes** refer to the effects of healthcare on the health status of patients and populations. Service output dimensions include patient satisfaction or patients' perception of quality, patient knowledge, attitudes, etc. Outcome measures are the ideal indicator and may seem to represent the "gold standard" in measuring quality, but are the most difficult to measure as it is the result of numerous factors, many beyond providers' control. The context (structure) in which care is delivered affects processes and outcomes. Structure and

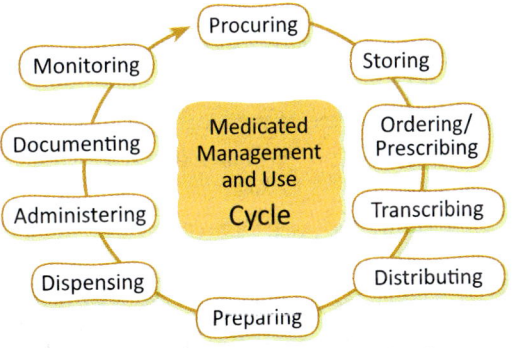

Roles and responsibility of a pharmacist

process are readily measured – (waiting time, waiting room was clean, the pharmacist was polite or not). The processes used in the various settings of pharmacy practice all comply with the same principles, although they may differ in application.

Given the typical nature of the pharmacist's role, process indicators are best suited to evaluate quality of the clinical pharmacist services. However, process indicators relevant to pharmacists' activities are not yet fully described in the literature. The framework is described below. Quality assurance processes of pharmaceutical care services serve to contribute towards better patient outcomes.

Definitions of the quality assurance of pharmaceutical care should encompass both technical standards and patients' expectations. While no single definition of health service quality applies in all situations, the following common definition is a helpful guide:

"Quality assurance is that set of activities that are carried out to monitor and improve performance so that the health care provided is as effective and as safe as possible".

Quality assurance can also be defined as "all activities that contribute to defining, designing, assessing, monitoring, and improving the quality of health care". These activities can be performed as part of the accreditation of pharmacies, supervision of pharmacy health workers, or other efforts to improve the performance and the quality of health services.

C. THE SIX DOMAINS OF HEALTHCARE QUALITY

It means providing care that does not vary in quality because of personal characteristics such as gender, ethnicity, geographic location or social-economic status. A handful of analytic frameworks for quality assessment have guided measure development initiatives in the public and private sectors. One of the most influential is the framework put forth by the Institute of Medicine (IOM), which includes the following six aims for the health care system:

Safe: Avoiding harm to patients from the care that is intended to help them.

Effective: Providing services based on scientific knowledge to all who could benefit and refraining from providing services to those not likely to benefit (avoiding under use and misuse, respectively).

Patient-centered: Providing care that is respectful of and responsive to individual patient preferences, needs, and values and ensuring that patient values guide all clinical decisions.

Timely: Reducing waits and sometimes harmful delays for both those who receive and those who give care.

Efficient: Avoiding waste, including waste of equipment, supplies, ideas, and energy.

Equitable: Providing care that does not vary in quality because of personal characteristics such as gender, ethnicity, geographic location, and socioeconomic status.

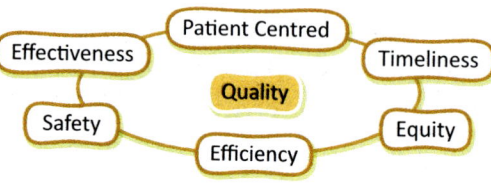

Six domains of health care quality

D. GOOD PHARMACY PRACTICE INDICATORS

Good Pharmacy Practice (GPP) indicators should cover five essential components (system, storage, services, dispensing and use) to assess standard requirements for pharmacy practices which are in line with most countries official licensing requirements. However, requirements and practice implementation may vary between countries.

1. Indicators to assess the availability and use of a prescribing recording system, degree of computerisation, and implementation of stock management and re-order system.

2. Storage indicators to assess presence of pests, cleanliness of the dispensing and storage area, pharmacy hygiene, storage conditions, system and practices.

3. Service indicators to assess prescription load, opening hours, staff availability and qualifications, availability of services, and tests and health promotion activities.

4. Dispensing indicators to assess information available to dispenser, product range, dispensing time, packaging material, dispensing equipment, dispensing procedure and contact with prescribers.

5. Rational use indicators to assess information available or provided to patients, patient care, labelling, and rational prescribing. Communication and the involvement of patient & carers

in the treatment is an integral component of effective pharmacy services. Patients (and/or carers) should have access to information & support in order to empower patients to make informed choices about the use of medicines or the implication of choosing not to take them.

Examples of evidence:

1. Patient Information:
   i. Patients are given written information on their medication & how to use them. Patient information leaflet (PILs) are available for all medicines.
   ii. Ward staff are trained to ensure that patients are not discharged without seeing a pharmacists and patient gets a PIL.
2. Pharmacists contact helpline is available e.g., advertised on PIL, discharge document, prescription, website, etc.
3. Pharmacy support:
   i. Ward staff refers patient to pharmacy, if patient need additional medicines support.
   ii. Health promotion and well being services- sign posting to smoking cessaton and alcohol withdrawal services.
4. High-alert or High-risk medicines: checklists for all these medicines are available and pharmacists and ward-staff are trained to use them.
5. Adherence to medicines
   i. Medication reconciliation
   ii. Polypharmacy
   iii. STOPP[3] and START – tools to simplify patient's medicines. STOPP and START criteria provide rules of avoidance of potentially inappropriate prescribing and potential prescribing omissions in elderly age group and improve medication appropriateness.

E. CLINICAL PHARMACY'S KEY PERFORMANCE INDICATORS (KPIs)

Pharmacy leaders and hospital administrators are charged with ensuring that pharmacists provide the best care for patients within a given budget, thus supporting the effective use of health care resources. Key performance indicators are quantifiable measures of quality that can be used to track an organization's progress toward achieving intended goals related to process inputs, process outputs, or outcomes. In other words the KPIs are a snap shot in time. Pharmacy managers may use KPI data to evaluate and enhance patient care activities.

Key performance indicators differ from workload measurement or workload management because they are selected on the basis of a proven association with a positive patient outcome, whereas workload measurement or management counts the frequency of an activity that is not necessarily specifically known to affect outcomes for individual patients. Process measurement, such as counting the number of patients who have received specific KPI activities in relation to the total number of patients, can elevate the professional accountability of the pharmacists and provide recognition for their work.

---

3. STOPP is the screening tool of older people's prescriptions as some drugs are potentially inappropriate for elderly patients and START is the screening tool to alert to right treatment (START) criteria.

Clinical Pharmacy Key Performance Indicators (KPIs)[4]

KPI	Description
Medication reconciliation[5] on admission, transition point[6]	Proportion of patients who receive documented admission medication reconciliation (as well as resolution of identified discrepancies) performed by a pharmacist completed within 24h/72h
Medication reconciliation at discharge	Proportion of patients who receive documented discharge medication reconciliation and resolution of identified discrepancies by a pharmacist
Pharmaceutical care plan	Proportion of patients for whom pharmacists have developed/initiated a pharmaceutical care plan
Drug therapy problems	Number of drug therapy problems addressed by a pharmacist per admission; Number of medicines information queries completed
Inter-professional patient care or medical rounds	Proportion of patients for whom pharmacists participate in inter-professional patient care rounds to improve medication management
Dispensing errors	Number of actual dispensing errors reported or number of dispensing errors prevented (near misses); percentage of charts with level 2 pharmacy checks carried out; number of complaints
Patient education during hospital stay	Proportion of patients who receive education from a pharmacist about their disease(s) and medications(s) during their hospital stay
Patient education at discharge	Proportion of patients who receive medication education about side effects, precautions, etc. by a pharmacist at discharge
Bundled patient care interventions	Proportion of patients who receive comprehensive direct patient care from a pharmacist working in collaboration with the health care team

III. INFORMATION MANAGEMENT AND THE USE OF EVIDENCE

Medicines can be one of the most cost-effective interventions in health care systems in terms of alleviating pain, suffering and even preventing death. In addition, they can contribute to savings of limited health care resources. However, the marketing practices used by many pharmaceutical companies make it very difficult to identify real improvements in the field of pharmaceuticals. It is, therefore, essential for pharmacists to understand and be able to use the tools of critical appraisal and cost-

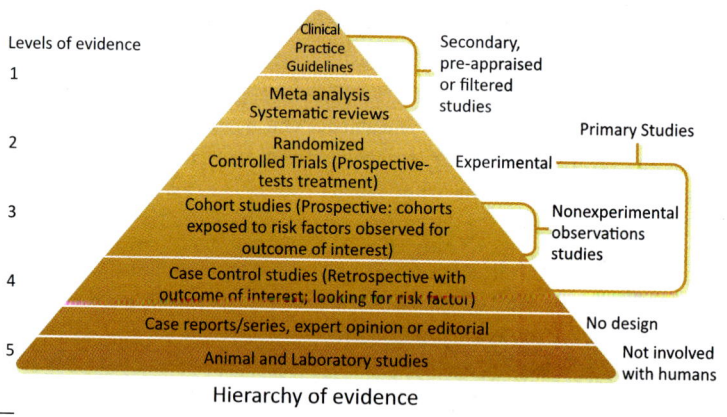

Hierarchy of evidence

---

4   Adapted from Measurement of Clinical Pharmacy Key Performance Indicators to Focus and Improve Your Hospital Pharmacy Practice Elaine Lo, Daniel Rainkie, William M Semchuk, Sean K Gorman, Kent Toombs, Richard S Slavik, David Forbes, Andrea Meade, Olavo Fernandes, and Sean P Spina. CJHP – Vol. 69, , No. 2 – March–April 2016; 149-155.

5   Medication reconciliation is a formal process for creating the most complete and accurate list possible of a patient's current medications and comparing the list to those in the patient record or medication orders.

6   Transition point refers to the various points where a patient moves to, or returns from, a particular physical location or makes contact with a health care professional for the purposes of receiving health care. This includes transitions between home, hospital, residential care settings and consultations with different health care providers in out-patient facilities.

effectiveness analysis as they evaluate the huge amount of information that reaches them. They should also share their critical appraisals with other health care professionals, notably prescribers. The techniques used have been incorporated in the emerging disciplines of evidence-based medicine/pharmacotherapy and pharmaco-economics.

Evidence-based medicine (EBM) attempts to move practice and prescribing away from a circumstantial and anecdotal approach to a reliance on the best possible evidence for the effectiveness of a medicine or procedure. What EBM aims to do is to integrate the best research evidence with clinical expertise and patient values. The process applied in assessing clinical evidence is termed "critical appraisal".

In many cases, however, practitioners do not have access to "best evidence" because of the circumstances in which they practice. In such cases, an approach often used is to develop specific prescribing guidelines. In this way the number of choices is restricted to those which are expected to produce the best possible results, particularly in resource limited environments. The relevant evidence is used to develop standard treatment guidelines, protocols or clinical guidelines to assist the process of decision-making and to contribute to rational and cost-effective health care.

The following section aims to provide the pharmacist with information about ways to keep up-to-date with changes in information, legislation, training and outcomes methods. It also provides an overview of drug information resources available and provides guidelines for interpreting and evaluating these and other information sources.

A. SOURCES OF MEDICINES INFORMATION

Numerous resources of medicines information are available, including, drug compendia, national medicines lists, essential medicines and treatment guidelines, drug formularies, drug bulletins, medical journals, drug information centres, reference books, information on internet and information provided by the pharmaceutical industry. Numerous reference books exist on a wide range of topics. It is, therefore, important to evaluate the quality of each publication. The frequency of new editions is an important criterion in choosing reference books. Only publications that are revised every two to five years can provide up-to-date knowledge. Even then they are not fully up-to-date since considerable time is needed to complete the different phases of writing, editing and publishing the books.

Reference books that cover general pharmacology are *Goodman and Gilman's: the Pharmacological Basis of Therapeutics* whereas *Lippincott's Illustrated Reviews* by Sangeeta Sharma & Valpandian; *The Pharmacological Basis of Therapeutics* and *Clinical Pharmacology* by Laurence are examples of text books on pharmacotherapy. *Applied Pharmacokinetics: Principles of Therapeutic Drug Monitoring* by Evans et al. provides information on pharmacokinetics and therapeutic drug monitoring. *Hansten and Horn's Drug Interactions Analysis and Management* is a primary source for information on drug interactions. In addition, *Martindale's The Complete Drug Reference* and National Formulary of India, the *American Hospital Formulary* Service (AHFS) *Drug Information* and *British National Formulary (BNF)* provide detailed drug information on a wide range of medicines.

1. Drug compendia

Drug compendia vary in scope and content and are published in many countries. Compendia usually include generic and brand names, chemical composition, indications and contraindications, warnings, precautions and interactions, side-effects, administration and dosing guidelines. Some compendia like the *Physician's Desk Reference* in the USA are based on official labelling information for the product as proved by the regulatory authority. Others like the *Monthly Index of Medical*

Specialities (MIMS) are commercially sponsored. The *United States Pharmacopeia Dispensing Information (USP DI)* and the *British National Formulary (BNF)* (http://www.bnf.org/) are comprehensive and objective compendia and provide information on comparative assessments, as well as criteria for choice within well-defined therapeutic categories.

2. National lists of Essential Medicines, Treatment Guidelines and Drug Formularies

National lists of essential medicines with or without Standard Treatment Guidelines exist in many developing countries. These lists are based on consensus of what are the most common diseases and complaints and define the range of medicines that should be available for a specific level of care. The pharmacist should verify whether such treatment guidelines exist in their health facility and try to obtain the most recent edition. If no national/state/hospital list of essential medicines is available, the WHO Model List of Essential Medicines can be consulted. The WHO Model List, which is updated every two years, is available in print and electronic database at the WHO Essential Medicines Library. It includes data such as summaries of relevant WHO clinical guidelines, the most important systematic reviews, important references, indicative cost information, information on nomenclature, and quality assurance standards.

The *WHO Model Formulary* presents model formulary information for all medicines on the WHO Model List of Essential Medicines and provides a starting point for countries and health facilities wishing to develop their own national formularies. It is available in print, as well as at their web site.

National or institutional drug formularies are usually developed by Drugs and Therapeutic Committees (DTCs) and contain the list of medicines that are approved for use in a specific institution, district, region or country. In India, Indian National Formulary has been developed (Indian Pharmacopoeia) by Indian Pharmacopoeia Commission. In addition, many health insurance companies, hospitals, and care centres have their own formulary, listing the products that are reimbursed.

3. Drug bulletins

Drug bulletins can be a valuable source of information in keeping up-to-date. Many drug bulletins are not sponsored by the pharmaceutical industry and provide impartial assessment of medicines and practical recommendations based on comparison between treatment alternatives.

4. Journals

There is a wide range of journals available that can assist the pharmacist in keeping up-to-date in the different aspects of pharmaceutical practice. *Pharmacotherapy*, *The Annals of Pharmacotherapy* and *Expert Opinion on Pharmacotherapy* provide information on pharmacotherapy. The general medical journals such as the *Lancet*, the *New England Journal of Medicine*, the *British Medical Journal, etc.* provide information on patient care and pharmacotherapy. The *American Journal of Health-System Pharmacy* provides information on pharmacy in health systems and patient care. The *International Journal of Pharmacy Practice* is an example of a journal that focuses on pharmacy practice. Although good medical journals are peer-reviewed, do not assume that because a review article or research study appears in print it is necessarily a good science. Use the guidelines described in Section below to evaluate all materials.

5. Drug information centres

Before responding to any queries, the pharmacist should first ensure that the information obtained is reliable (see Section below on how to evaluate the medical literature). The purpose of drug information centre is to provide authentic individualized, accurate, relevant and unbiased drug information to the consumers and healthcare professionals regarding medication related inquiries for health care & drug safety aspects by answering their call regarding all the critical problems on drug information, their uses and their side effects. Apart from that the centre also provides in-depth, impartial source of crucial drug information to meet the needs of the practicing physicians, pharmacists and other health care professionals to safeguard the health, financial and legal interests of the patient & to broaden the pharmacists role visible in the society & community. Many countries have drug information centres and often these centres also provide information on poisons. For example, the UK Medicines Information Pharmacists Group provides medicines information on their web site at: http://www.druginfozone.org/.

In India, the Poison Information Centre at All India Institute of Medical Sciences (AIIMS) provides poison information round-the-clock to hospitals of Delhi and other parts of India. The Institute monitors adverse drugs reaction and reports to Uppsala monitoring center in Sweden. Other state drug information center also provide some amount of Poison information to their respective community.

List of Drug Information Centres Run at State Pharmacy Councils in India (Regional) is as follows:

1. CDMU Documentation Centre, Calcutta

2. Karnataka State Pharmacy Council (KSPC), Bangalore, Karnataka

3. JSS, Ooty,

4. Drug Information Center, Maharashtra State Pharmacy Council, Maharashtra

5. Pharma Information Center, Tamilnadu, Chennai

6. Andhra Pradesh State Pharmacy Council, Andhra Pradesh.

7. Drug Information Center, Jaipur, Rajasthan.

8. Drug Information Center, Raipur, Chhattisgarh.

The Pharmaceutical Clearing House and the Pan-American Pharmaceutical Forum, developed by the Pan American Health Organization (PAHO) and WHO, are also important references for obtaining drug information and for keeping up-to-date.

Other useful sites include the following:

1. WHO Essential Medicines Library: http://mednet3.who.int/EMLib/

2. Free Medical Journals site: http://www.freemedicaljournals.com which is dedicated to the promotion of free access to medical journals over the Internet.

3. Catalogue of Internet health resources with links to relevant sites http://www.bubl.ac.uk/link/med.html.

6. Retrieval (and evaluation) of medicines information online

Many medical articles are indexed in the Medline database, which is available in most medical and science libraries. Medline is compiled by the National Library of Medicine of the United States and indexes over 3800 journals published in over 70 countries. Free access to the Medline database is available through the Internet by using the following Internet address: http://www.ncbi.nlm.nih.gov/PubMed/. Articles can be traced by using any word listed in the database as keywords. The words listed in the database include words in the title, abstract, authors' names and the institution where the research was done. Other sites such as http://www.medscape.com/ or http://biomail.sourceforge.net/biomail/ can also be used to search for information.

It is essential to ensure that the data obtained online are reliable. The following points can be used to determine, if an article published on the Internet is authoritative:

1. What is the author's qualification for writing on the subject?
2. Is the author connected to an organization with an established reputation?
3. Look for the source. Is it a major university or institute specializing in that area?
4. Is it published on a reputable website? Has it been peer-reviewed?
5. Has the author taken care in formatting, logic, structure and development of the argument?
6. Does the article meet all the criteria as discussed in following section on evaluation of medical literature?

7. Information from a Pharmaceutical /Medical Representative ("medical rep")

The pharmaceutical industry has large budgets for promotion and uses many different channels of communication for promoting their products. However, commercial information often emphasizes only the positive aspects of the products. Because pharmacists are members of committees or groups that decide on a formulary or protocol, they are often subjected to promotional pressures by medical representatives. The pharmacist needs to be fully aware of the content of promotional materials in order to put forward a rational argument for the appropriate use of medicines. It is, therefore, important to take control of an appointment with a "medical rep" in order to obtain the less positive information as well.

The following guidelines may be used to obtain the most out of a visit by a "medical representative" or "drug representative":

1. See the "rep" only by appointment, determine the purpose of the visit in advance and confine the interview to that specific purpose only.
2. Take charge of the interview. Do not hear out a rehearsed sales routine but ask specific questions, especially about the adverse drug reactions and the therapeutic value of the product.
3. Request independent published evidence from reputable peer-reviewed journals.
4. Promotion brochures often contain unpublished material, misleading graphs and selective quotations. The pharmacist needs to appraise them so as to be able to deal with prescribers who have been influenced by the graphics and claims.
5. Ignore anecdotal "evidence" such as the fact that a medical celebrity or major institution is prescribing or using the product.
6. Request evidence by using the "STEP" analysis:
   i. *Safety* – the likelihood of long-term or serious side-effects caused by the product;
   ii. *Tolerability* – is best measured by comparing the pooled withdrawal rates between the product and its most significant competitor;
   iii. *Efficacy* – the most relevant dimension is how the product compares with your current favourite;
   iv. *Price* – direct plus indirect costs (cost of therapy and not cost of unit alone) should be taken into account.
7. Ask for copies of papers of any clinical trials used to support the company's argument.

8. Evaluate the evidence stringently, paying particular attention to the power (sample size) and methodological quality of clinical trials and the use of surrogate end points. Do not accept theoretical arguments in the product's favour without direct evidence that they translate into clinical benefit. Bear in mind that negative papers are unlikely to be quoted or referenced in the promotional literature or mentioned by the Rep.

9. Do an independent search of the literature.

10. Do not accept the newness of a product as an argument for changing to it. There are good scientific arguments for doing the opposite. A new medicine is not always better or safer.

11. Decline to try the product through starter packs or by participating in small-scale uncontrolled "research studies".

12. Record in writing the content of the interview and return to these notes, if the representative requests another meeting with you.

B. EVALUATION OF THE MEDICAL LITERATURE

As the number of publications describing new treatment options in health care increases, the need to evaluate the medical literature critically becomes even more important. It is only after a critical review that a pharmacist can derive valid conclusions and incorporate the information into pharmaceutical care and practice.

The following three questions will help you:

1. Why was the study done and what hypotheses were tested?

2. What type of study was done?

3. Was the study design appropriate for the purpose of the study?

   i. Most papers have a similar format, which includes the introduction, methods, results and discussion.

   ii. The Introduction should acquaint the reader with the problem statement and provide the necessary background to enable the reader to understand the problem and evaluate the outcome of the study. A well-defined study objective should also be stated in the Introduction.

   iii. The Methods section should be clear and detailed enough so that the reader could repeat the investigation. The study design and sample should be clear to the reader. The statistical methods used should be stated in the Methods.

   iv. A well-written Results section should present data on all subjects involved in the study including information on lost to follow-up patients and measured parameters as mentioned in the Methods.

   v. In the Discussion, the results are interpreted and related to, or compared with, previous work or practice. The reader should be aware of biased language and comments unjustified by the results. The reader should be aware that small differences in results may have been overemphasized by stating the differences in percentages. For example, if 5 out of 1000 patients experience an adverse effect on Medicine A and 10 out of 1000 on Medicine B the difference in experiencing adverse effects could be expressed as 50% more in Medicine B than Medicine A. In other words, the relative risk reduction (RRR) achieved using Medicine A rather than Medicine B is 50%, whereas the absolute risk reduction (ARR) is 0.5%.

Some commonly used definitions are shown in box below:

Some commonly used definitions in clinical trial reports

Randomized controlled trial (RCT)	Clinical trial where at least two treatment groups are compared. One must be a control group, e.g. receiving standard care or a placebo treatment. Allocation to a group must be random and unbiased.
Randomisation	Process of allocating individuals to the alternative treatments in a clinical trial, avoiding bias. Should produce groups which are similar, except for the treatment of interest.
Blinding	The process of ensuring that participants or researchers (single-blind) or participants and researchers (double-blind) are unaware of which treatment group participants have been randomized to, reducing the possibility of bias in the results.
Intention-to-treat analysis (ITT)	All patients allocated to one arm of a RCT are analysed in that arm, whether or not they completed the prescribed treatment/regimen.
Experimental event rate (EER)	Risk (or chance) of outcome event in experimental group. Control event rate (CER)-Risk (or chance) of outcome event in control group.
Relative risk or risk ratio (RR)	A measure of the chance of the event occurring in the experimental group relative to it occurring in the control group. RR = 1 means that exposure does not affect the outcome; RR < 1 means that the risk of the outcome is decreased by the exposure; RR > 1 means risk of the outcome is increased by the exposure.
Relative risk reduction (RRR)	The difference in the proportion of events between the control and experimental groups, relative to the proportion of events in the control group.
Absolute risk reduction (ARR)	The absolute difference between the risk of the event in the control and experimental groups.
Number needed to treat (NNT)	The number of patients who needed to be treated to prevent the occurrence of one adverse event (e.g. complication, death) or promote the occurrence of one beneficial event (e.g. cessation of smoking).
Confidence interval	For whatever effect being measures (e.g. RR, RRR, ARR, NTT) the confidence interval is the range of values within which the "true" value in the population is found. Generally expressed as a 95% confidence interval, i.e. you can be 95% confident that the population value lies within those limits

The evidence-based approach turns clinical and economic problems into questions, followed by a systematic literature search and comprehensive analysis to inform decisions.

SUMMARY OF BASIC CRITERIA FOR CRITICAL APPRAISAL OF STUDIES ON THERAPY

1. Key factors– the study addresses a clear focused question. Clearly states– Patients, intervention, comparison, and outcome
2. Assignment of Patients - whether randomized, controlled
3. Did the study used valid methods to address the question
4. Is study important
5. Accountability of study participants– all subjects who entered the trial accounted at its conclusion
6. Were they analysed in the groups to which they were randomized e.g. intention-to-treat (INT) analysis
7. Blinding-Whether patients and doctors were blind to which treatment was being received
8. Beside from the experimental treatment, were the groups treated equally; in continuation

9. Are the valid results of this study important. Determine relevance of study results

10. Are these valid results applicable to my patient or population

11. Treatment effect– in experimental control group

12. Determine applicability of study results in respect of

   i. Patient's characteristics

   ii. Feasibility of treatment as it relates to setting

   iii. Benefits and harms

   iv. Patient's preferences

If answer to any of the above question is 'no' save the trouble of reading the rest of the promotional material

13. How large was the treatment effect & how results were expressed (RRR; NNT, etc.).

14. How precise were the results– Whether results presented with confidence interval.

15. The following questions assist the process of moving through these steps:

   i. Does the medicine of interest have any therapeutic advantages over a currently used product?

   ii. Does the medicine of interest have any safety advantages over the currently used product?

If the answer to these questions is no, then the matter should not be pursued, and the current/ comparator product should continue to be used. For the pharmacist in the patient care setting, the question would be asked in terms of verifying the decision made by the prescriber: is the medicine prescribed the best choice related to the indication?

The process of "systematic review" of the literature can be applied to answer these questions. Systematic review may be supported by a technique known as meta-analysis in some cases. A systematic review is the process of systematically locating, appraising and synthesizing evidence from scientific studies in order to obtain a reliable overview. Systematic reviews are distinct from traditional literature reviews in that they are based on a strict scientific design to minimize bias and ensure reliability. Best evidence is based on selecting appropriate study types and evaluating the methodological quality of the studies.

C. ADHERENCE TO TREATMENT AND THE PATIENT'S VIEWPOINT

To use evidence in improving health care, the viewpoint of the patient is very important. The beliefs, values, preferences, concerns and economic situation of patients have a direct effect on their perceptions of the possible benefits and harms of, their acceptance of, and their adherence to specific treatment modalities and/or drug regimens. The applicability to an individual patient is always the final step in the appraisal of evidence for therapy. The patient's characteristics, the feasibility of treatment as it relates to setting, benefits and harms, and the patient's own preferences all need to be taken into account. The selected strategy should be agreed with the patient; this agreement on outcome, and how it may be achieved, is termed concordance. Concordance is an important factor for adherence to therapy.

As far as patient-related factors for adherence are concerned, women tend to be more adherent than men, younger patients and the very elderly are less adherent, and people living alone are less adherent than those with family, partners or spouses. Specific education interventions have been shown to improve adherence. Patient characteristics such as illiteracy, poor eyesight or cultural attitudes (e.g., preference for traditional or alternative medicines and suspicion of modern medicine) may be very important in some individuals or societies. Such attitudes need to be discussed, brought out into the open and addressed. Other factors which influence adherence may be linked to the prescriber/practitioner and his/her relationship with the patient, the health condition, the prescription, the pharmacist or the health system. A good patient-practitioner relationship is crucial to concordance.

"Satisfaction with the interview" on the part of the patient has been consistently shown to be one of the highest predictors of good adherence. Conditions with a severe prognosis (e.g., cancer) or painful conditions (e.g., rheumatoid arthritis) elicit better adherence rates than asymptomatic, "perceived as benign" conditions such as hypertension, or conditions which occur at long intervals, such as epilepsy. Prescriptions for many medications or for more than two doses per day tend to decrease adherence, as do adverse effects, which patients may not always mention. The pharmacist's personality and professional manner is important, especially when generic medicines are substituted for brand name medicines.

The healthcare system may be the biggest hindrance of all to adherence. Long waiting times, uncaring staff, uncomfortable environments, exhausted drug supplies and long distances between the patient and the healthcare facility can all have a major impact on adherence.

1. Causes of non-compliance/non-adherence

There are many possible reasons for noncompliance and sometimes there are valid reasons for poor adherence:

- The patient suffers adverse effects
- The patient does not think the drug is effective
- The patient forgets to take the drug
- The patient believes the disease is cured because the symptoms have abated
- The patient has misunderstood the user instructions
- The patient has run out of the drug
- The patient does not master the administration technique, e.g. inhalation
- The drug formulation is unsuitable or drug is unacceptable, e.g. unpleasant taste
- The patient uses many drugs simultaneously (polypharmacy)
- Frequent dosages
- The patient has other objections towards the use of a certain drug.

2. Situations where compliance / non-adherence is important

There are several situations where compliance is of even greater importance than normal:

- When using drugs with a narrow therapeutic range (such as phenytoin, carbamazepines, lithium, gentamicin).
- When using drugs that may produce serious adverse effects (e.g. cytotoxics, immunosuppressives and anticoagulants).
- With hormone supplementation (e.g. metabolic disease, diabetes, adrenal failure).
- In the treatment of glaucoma and epilepsy.
- In the treatment of certain infections, e.g. when treating tuberculosis, multidrug-resistant tuberculosis, AIDS.

3. The interventions for improving adherence rates

These may be classified into the following categories:

- Staff motivation and supervision—includes training and management processes aimed at improving the way in which providers care for patients.

- Defaulter action—the action to be taken when a patient fails to keep a pre-arranged appointment e.g., DOTS clinic.

- Prompts—routine reminders for patients to keep pre-arranged appointments.

- Health education—provision of information about the disease and the need to attend for treatment.

- Incentives and reimbursements—money or cash or in kind to reimburse the expenses of attending the treatment centre, or to improve the attractiveness of visiting the treatment centre.

- Peer assistance—people from the same social group helping someone with the disease such as tuberculosis to return to the health centre by prompting or accompanying him or her.

- Directly observed therapy (DOT)—an identified, trained and supervised agent (health worker, community volunteer or family member) directly monitors patients swallowing their medicines as one of a range of measures to promote adherence e.g., TB treatment.

4. Patient Charters and Patient Responsibilities have been established to accommodate patients' rights. These charters have certain common features concerning the ways in which patients should be treated, however, at the same time, patients also have responsibilities:

Patient's rights

- To receive safe, quality and effective medicines
- To be advised and counselled on the appropriate use of medicines
- To receive the right medicine in the right quantity
- To be treated with dignity
- To be seen by a pharmacist who can be identified by name
- To be assured of confidentiality about their illness and treatment
- To receive pharmaceutical services in a pharmacy which complies with good pharmacy practice standards
- To expect the highest degree of honesty from their pharmacist in dealing with their medical expenses and funding
- To feel able to complain or express a need
- To participate in decision-making on matters affecting their health and their medicine
- To get a second opinion.

Patient's responsbility

- To be reasonable and courteous
- To assist their pharmacist in complying with legal requirements relating to medicine use
- To use medicine with care
- To report any problems experienced with their medicine.
- It is essential that patients are informed about their options when faced with dealing with their illness. These options can be clarified by the responses to a small number of questions.

2 | Good Dispensing Practices

Pharmacist must ensure that all medicines and scheduled substances are procured, stored, dispensed or supplied from a pharmacy in accordance with the relevant law's such as Drugs and Cosmetics Act, Narcotic Drugs & Psychotropic Substance (NDPS) Act, Pharmacy Practice Regulations. The storage, dispensing or supply of any medicine or scheduled substance by a pharmacist, or pharmacist intern may only take place in or from a pharmacy that complies with relevant good pharmacy practice guidelines relating to premises, equipment, reference sources and safety and is duly recorded in terms of the relevant Acts as applicable.

Guidelines for the dispensing of medicine or scheduled substances in the following sections apply on the prescription of an authorized prescriber.

I. DISPENSING CYCLE

The following phases are performed during the "dispensing" process: evaluation of the prescription, the preparation and labeling of the medicine prescribed and the advising of the patient, to ensure the optimal use of medicine.

1. The dispensing procedure must ensure that the prescriber's intentions are accurately interpreted, that the medicine is correctly dispensed with reasonable promptness and accuracy that an appropriate container and correct label are used. If, on occasion, a prescription cannot be dispensed, the patient must be advised of an alternative dispensing source or be referred back to the prescriber.

2. Within this procedure, physical and human resources should be allocated to ensure that prescriptions are dispensed safely and efficiently, with effective, interruption-free personal communication with the patient when that is considered necessary.

A. DISPENSING PROCEDURES

This section applies to pharmacists, pharmacist interns, pharmacist's assistants (post-basic) and other healthcare professional who are licensed to dispense and must be read and applied in context of its relevance and pertinence to the respective health care professional.

The dispensing process is divided into 3 phases, namely:

Phase 1: Evaluation of the prescription.

Phase 2: Preparation and labeling of the prescribed medicine.

Phase 3: Advising the patient to ensure the optimal use of medicine.

Phases 1 and 3 are performed by the pharmacist; in case performed by the pharmacist intern it should be under the supervision of the pharmacist to ensure the quality and safe use of medicine.

Phase 2, which involves the logistical and manipulative functions, may be performed by a Pharmacist's assistant (post-basic) under the supervision of a pharmacist.

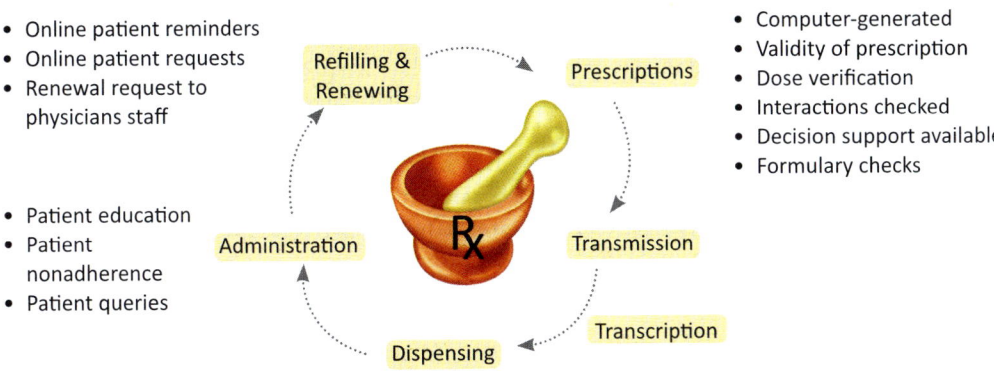

- Online patient reminders
- Online patient requests
- Renewal request to physicians staff

Refilling & Renewing

Prescriptions

- Computer-generated
- Validity of prescription
- Dose verification
- Interactions checked
- Decision support available
- Formulary checks

- Patient education
- Patient nonadherence
- Patient queries

Administration

Transmission

Transcription

Dispensing

Phase 1: Evaluation of the prescription

1. Reception of the prescription and confirmation of the integrity of this written communication. Adequate procedures should exist for:

   i. Identifying the patient, and the prescriber.

   ii. Ensuring the legality/authenticity of the prescription.

   iii. Interpreting the type of treatment and the prescriber's intentions.

   iv. Identifying the medicine, and checking the pharmaceutical form, strength, appropriate dosage, presentation, method of administration and duration of treatment.

   v. Informing the patient of the benefits of the substitution for a branded medicine of an interchangeable generic medicine, whenever applicable.

   vi. Helping the patient to resolve the problem when the prescription cannot be dispensed.

2. Assessment of the prescription to ensure the optimal use of medicine. Each prescription should be professionally assessed by a pharmacist on:

   i. Therapeutic aspects (pharmaceutical and pharmacological) i.e. the safety of the medicine; possible contra-indications; drug/drug interactions; drug/disease interactions; treatment duplications;

   ii. Appropriateness for the individual; and

   iii. Social, legal and economic aspects.

3. Pharmacist intervention - Whenever necessary the pharmacist should communicate with the prescriber regarding any identified problems and work out a plan of action with the prescriber and/or the patient.

4. For the assessment of a prescription the following can be used:

   i. Questions put to the patient or caregiver;

   ii. Questions put to the prescriber where doubts arise or further information is required;

   iii. Pharmacopoeias, formularies, technical books, electronic sources, professional journals, compendia of pharmaceutical legislation and medicine supply agreements with the health services; and

   iv. Outside information from drug information centres, competent authorities and pharmaceutical manufacturers.

Phase 2: Preparation and labelling of the prescribed medicine

Selecting or preparing the medicine includes the following activities:

1. Patient-ready-packs/pre-packed medicines are correctly selected.

2. Preparation of extemporaneous preparations[7] when required. Every pharmacy should have adequate facilities for dispensing individual prescriptions extemporaneously. e.g., dermatological & eye dosage forms, oral formulations, suspensions that are not commercially available. Tablets are cut into halves or quarters to obtain appropriately sized dosage unit for children. Pharmacists need to have access to stability, compatibility and formulation information as well as appropriate training to ensure that the patients are supplied high quality, safe, and effective preparation.

3. Counting must be done on a clean counting tray and the final dosage form placed in a suitable container.

4. The container of the medicine must be clearly labeled with the correct directions along with any other information for the safe, proper and effective use of the medicine. Cautionary/advisory labels and instructions must always be used. See section on labels and auxiliary labels.

5. All dispensing procedures must be carefully checked for accuracy and completeness.

6. Signing the prescription. Accountability must be accepted by the pharmacist who signs the prescription or copy of the prescription accepting liability for the correctness of the dispensing of the medicine and confirming that the medicine was supplied.

Phase 3: Advising of the patient to ensure the safe and efficacious use of medicine

1. Advising a patient or the patient's agent/caregiver (physical presence is preferred) should be carried out by a pharmacist.

2. A patient information leaflet, containing the information as prescribed as per hospital policy must be made available at the point of dispensing.

3. Additional advice in writing should accompany the medicine, whenever required.

4. Information should be structured to meet the needs of individual patients.

For details see section on Patient education and Counseling

Standard drug information for consumers in Patient Information Leaflets (PILs)

1. *Standard drug information for consumers*

2. What is _____ (insert product name)?

3. Why use _____ ?

4. When should _____ be/not be used?

5. What precautions should be taken?

   i.   By children

   ii. During pregnancy

   iii. When breast feeding

   iv. While driving or operating machinery

   v.   If taking other medicines

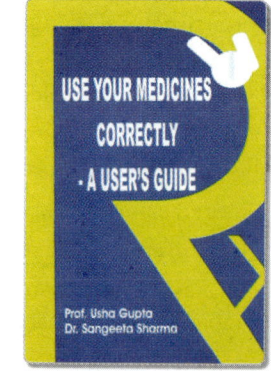

---

7 An extemporeneous preparation is a drug specially prepared by a pharmacist because an appropriate dosage of the medicine is not commercially available.

6. How should I take _____ ?

7. What should I do if I miss a dose?

8. What should I do if I take too many tablets?

9. What undesirable effect might _____ cause?

10. How should I store _____ ?

Monitoring patient outcomes

Monitoring patient outcomes includes the ongoing evaluation of the patient and the therapeutic plan with regard to progress towards the therapeutic goal.

1. The pharmacist should assess the patient for signs of compliance, effectiveness and safety of the therapy.

2. The pharmacist should identify areas for modification, implementation of modifications (taking into account legal requirements), revise the patient record and record the action taken.

B. PROBLEMS AND ISSUES IN DISPENSING

1. Dispensing must be done under the supervision of a pharmacist.

2. In a pharmacy with only one pharmacist present, this pharmacist must be able to supervise activities in the medicines dispensing/sale area at the same time.

3. A pharmacist responsible for supervising the dispensing, sale or supply of any medicine in a pharmacy bears the associated legal and professional responsibility.

4. Every prescription for a medicine must be seen by a pharmacist and a judgment made by him/her as to what action is necessary.

5. The pharmacist must exercise judgment to ensure fulfillment of professional duties to the patients in the best possible way. The pharmacist must thus be able to delegate to pharmacist's assistants (post-basic) "phase 2" tasks that he/she is confident can be undertaken by them. The pharmacist must be available in the pharmacy to intervene, to advise and to check the dispensing of any prescription under his/her supervision.

6. Systems must be developed to ensure that the distribution of medicines is reliable and secure to the point of delivery.

7. Although collection and delivery of prescription should be avoided, however, if sometimes necessary, the best pharmaceutical service is provided where the opportunity exists for direct face-to face and one-on-one contact between patient and pharmacist.

8. In cases of uncertainty, the pharmacist must make every effort to contact the prescriber. If it is impossible to contact the prescriber, the pharmacist should use his/her professional judgment and decide, in all the circumstances, what course of action would be in the best interest of the patient.

9. Where the problem cannot be resolved and if there appears to be a potential risk to the patient, the pharmacist may decide not to dispense the prescription even if the prescriber confirms that the product should be dispensed. In taking this decision, however, the pharmacist should assess the relative harm, which may result from this refusal and use his/her professional judgment to decide what course of action would be in the best interest of the patient.

10. The prescription should be endorsed according to any action taken e.g. telephonic confirmation of an unusual dosage, etc.

11. **Forged prescriptions:** A pharmacist must be aware of the probable methods of prescription forgery and exercise due care to satisfy himself/herself that prescriptions are genuine.

12. **Individual Patient Prescription:** Medications should be dispensed in original container or individually labeled prescription containers. The amount of drug dispensed should be determined by hospital policy. Medication containers should not be altered by anyone other than pharmacy personnel.

C. LABELS

1. Labeling of dispensed products must be clear and legible and indelible; lettering must as far as possible be mechanically printed. Errors may be caused by poor labeling; optimize pharmacy computer-generated labeling and production of medication administration records.

2. Pharmacists should use standardized terminology, metric units, and generic nomenclature of all drug labels to minimize confusion. Exclude nonessential information from labels and reports. There should be a list of abbreviations and symbols approved by the Pharmacy and Therapeutics Committee.

3. Medication labels should be typed or machine printed and should be free from erasures and strikeovers. The labels should be firmly affixed to the container.

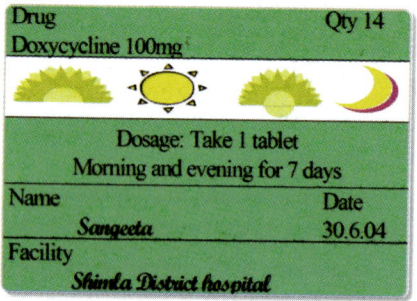
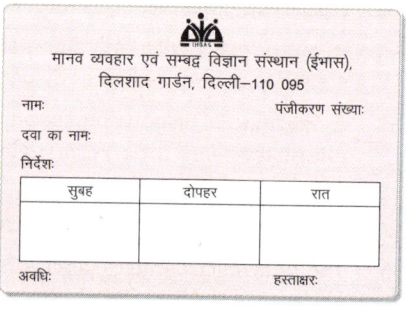

4. Syringe admixture labels

   i. Standardization of the way labels are placed on syringes can reduce errors.

   ii. Use of "For Oral Use Only" labels on oral syringes.

   iii. Placement of labels on IV bags

   iv. Warning labels for special parenterals such as:

   Vinca alkaloids, other antineoplastics

   Medications with specific infusion rates.

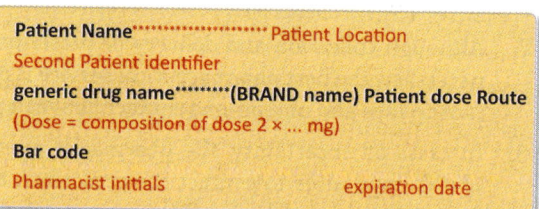

5. Computer order entry involves the selection of the correct medication, dosage strength, dosage form, quantity, directions for use, number of refills, and prescriber name. All of these parameters should be included on the label. If possible, the purpose of the medication should be printed on the dispensing label. Including the purpose on the label provides the patient with an additional means to verify and distinguish among their prescriptions.

6. Children pose a unique set of risks of medication errors, predominantly because of the need for dosage calculations, which are individually based on the patient's weight, age or body surface area, and their condition and improper oral liquid medications administration because of

misunderstandings with reading and labeling of oral syringes or use of such devices by parents of paediatric patients. Label should include warning to keep all medicines out of the reach of children. For details see following section on dispensing in special situations to children.

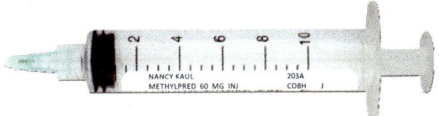

Properly labeled syringe for inpatient

D. DISPENSING CONTAINERS

1. The container must be appropriate for the product dispensed, bearing in mind the need to protect the product from moisture and sunlight as well as from mechanical stresses imparted by transport and use of the product.

2. All containers intended for medicinal products must be protected and kept free from contamination.

3. All solid dose oral preparations should be dispensed in a reclosable container or in original unit packaging of strips or blister type without cutting unless:

    i.   The original pack is such as to make this inadvisable/indispensable;

    ii. The patient is elderly or handicapped and will have difficulty in opening the reclosable container; or

    iii. A specific request is made that the product should not be dispensed in a reclosable container.

4. Advice must be given to keep all medicines out of the reach of children.

5. Reuse of containers

    i.   Plastic containers and caps for solid or liquid dose preparations must not be reused as satisfactory cleaning cannot be ensured.

    ii. Under no circumstances may reclosable child resistant closures be used more than once, as continued use affects the child resistant properties of the closure.

    iii. Glass containers are capable of being reused only after satisfactory cleaning and drying. High standards must be maintained, which may make reuse uneconomical.

II. MEDICATION SYSTEM

A. UNIT-DOSE MEDICATION SYSTEM

1. Unit-dose systems dispense medications contained in, and administered from, unit-dose packages and avoids the need for strip cutting. e.g., Single dose packing of albendazole and fluconazole should be dispensed as these medicines are administered as a single dose.

2. Supply of unit dose medication to the acute patient care area should be as per hospital policy.

3. The medication profile, if available, should be utilized for the individual medication doses to be scheduled, prepared, distributed and administered on a timely basis.

4. Unit-dose carts or medication trays should be used as medication storage facilities on the ward. The particular tray for a specific patient should be labeled with the patient's name, location and hospital number. The following information should be indicated on the individual dosage package:

    i.   Name of drug

    ii. Strength

    iii. Expiry date

    iv. Lot number

B. CONTROLLED DOSAGE SYSTEM

1. Medications should be dispensed in individually-labeled controlled dosage cards/containers.
2. The system should be designed so that each dose is designated for a specific time of administration.
3. The amount of the drug dispensed should be determined by hospital policy.
4. The processing of emergency "stat" orders should be determined through written hospital policy.

The pharmacist should exercise professional judgment at completion of the dispensing procedure to ensure the right drug is dispensed for administration to the right patient, in the right dose, via the right route, at the right time.

III. PATIENT COUNSELLING AND EDUCATION

Patients should consume medicines as prescribed by the doctor and this can only be ensured if the patient is educated and empowered to appropriate use of medicines. It is often seen that patient is neither provided adequate information by the doctor, nor by the pharmacist. Hence, many times patients either consume less medicine or more medicines. Either way it is harmful and unsafe for the patient.

A pharmacist should promote the safe and effective use of medication by educating patients about their drug therapy. *Most dispensing errors can be discovered during patient counseling and corrected before the patient leaves the pharmacy.*

Educating the patients about health:
1. Promotes healthy living
2. Prevents or minimizes disease
3. Increases adherence to treatment
4. Impacts/positive health outcomes

Common causes of non-compliance
1. Inappropriate attitudes and poor communication skills of providers
2. Patients' fear of asking questions
3. Inadequate consulting and dispensing time
4. Lack of access to printed information in simple language- Patient information leaflets (PIL) and adequate labels
5. Inability to pay for prescribed drugs
6. Complexity of drug regimen and long duration of treatment

Dispensing errors caused by poor patient education
1. Failure to adequately educate patients
2. Lack of pharmacist involvement in direct patient education
3. Failure to provide patients with understandable written instructions
4. Lack of involving patients in check systems
5. Not listening to patients when therapy is questioned or concerns are expressed

Communication and patient safety

1. Ineffective communication is reported as a significant contributing factor in medical errors and inadvertent patient harm. It is also the frequently cited category of root causes of sentinel events.

2. Effective communication, which is timely, accurate, complete, unambiguous, and understood by the recipient, reduces errors and results in improved patient safety.

3. Communication is the key to improve patient safety.

4. Non verbal communication constitutes most of the communication such as eye contact, facial expressions, body language, tone of voice, emphasis, deliberate silence, timing, appearance, touch, hand movements, etc.

Ways to Improve Listening Skills are:

- Stop talking
- Teach yourself to concentrate
- Take time to listen
- Listen with your eyes
- Listen to what is being said, not only how it is being said
- Suspend judgment
- Do not interrupt the speaker
- Remove distractions
- Listen for both feeling and content.
- Listen to the patient
- Encourage patient to ask questions
- Ask patients "Do you have any questions" Praise patients for asking questions
- "I am glad that you asked that question..."
- "Good question..."
- Answer all questions thoughtfully and carefully

Guidelines for the furnishing of information and advice

1. The responsible pharmacist must ensure that patients are counseled prior to discharge or transfer from hospital or when they are to be treated as outpatients.

2. The responsible pharmacist should ensure that only suitably experienced and trained staff carry out this task.

3. The pharmacist involved should assess each patient's ability to understand information imparted by question and answer and be able to modify their approach accordingly. Care should be taken with the advising of parents, relatives, the elderly or ethnic groups or where understanding is likely to be a problem.

4. The provision of advice should take place in a suitable environment and the patient should be put at ease, especially with regard to sensitive information. No information may be divulged about the affairs of any person obtained in the course of dispensing a prescription except to a person authorized to have access to such information and acting within his/her lawful jurisdiction.

5. Particular caution may be necessary when dealing with certain categories of patients, e.g. those attending addiction or venereal disease clinics.

6. Empower patient: Doctor should adequately explain the patient about each drug after writing the prescription and pharmacist should provide information either verbal or written at the time of dispensing. Minimum information that should be imparted during patient counseling should include the following:

   i. How to take each medicine, viz. dose, time, frequency, route and duration.

   ii. Specific precautions to be taken, viz. before or after meals, concurrent medications and food interaction.

   iii.   What adverse effects can be expected and when to report to the doctor?

   iv.   How medicines should be stored at home?

   v.   What to do, if a dose is missed?

   vi.   How to use devices such as MDI, Rotahaler

7. Patient should be told to inform the doctor about allergy to medicines and medicines they are already consuming for other diseases.

8. Review and repeat instructions regularly.

9. Make use of medicines organizers

10. Make use of printed information-adherence to treatment may be increased by the availability of printed information in simple language.

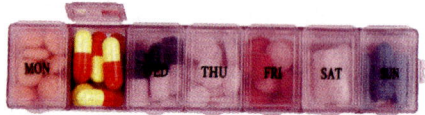

11. Public access to sources of impartial drug information is particularly important in view of increasing consumer participation in health care delivery.

IV. DISPENSING IN SPECIAL SITUATIONS

1. More detailed advice is especially important when certain drugs are supplied and in certain circumstances. Examples include:

   i.   Medicines that can sedate

   ii.   Medicines that have a narrow therapeutic index (e.g., antiepileptic medicines, lithium, gentamicin, cyclosporine)

   iii.   Unusual dose forms (e.g. fentanyl patches)

   iv.   Unusual frequency of use (e.g. alendronate, methotrexate)

   v.   When a new medicine is prescribed

   vi.   When there is a change in the dose or frequency of administration

   vii.   When the brand of medicine has changed

   viii.   When the medicine is a narcotic and psychotropic drug

   ix.   With each supply of medicine for which there are valid reasons for regular reinforcement of information (e.g. teratogenics or cytotoxics; major contraindications; special patient needs, such as language preference, vision, hearing or cognitive impairment, or cultural issues)

   x.   At regular intervals (e.g. six monthly) for medicines used for long-term therapy

   xi.   When the medicine is for a special population;

   xii.   If the patient is taking many medicines

   viii.   When there is an acute illness or event (e.g. hospital admission).

2. Dispensing to special populations

   The presence of certain life circumstances or comorbid medical or psychosocial conditions warrant special attention during treatment and dispensing such as in:

- Children
- Pregnancy & Lactation
- Disabilities in children
- Elderly
- Psychiatric disorders

A. CHILDREN

1. Unless the age is specified, the term 'child' includes persons aged 12 years and younger.

2. Children are not small adults.

3. Special care is needed in the neonatal period (first 30 days of life) in choosing drugs. Doses also should always be calculated with care. At this age, the risk of toxicity is increased by inefficient renal filtration, relative enzyme deficiencies, differing target organ sensitivity, and inadequate detoxifying systems causing delayed excretion.

4. Choose appropriate drug measuring device for liquid preparations. For a liquid oral preparation for doses smaller than 2.5 ml, an oral syringe be used.

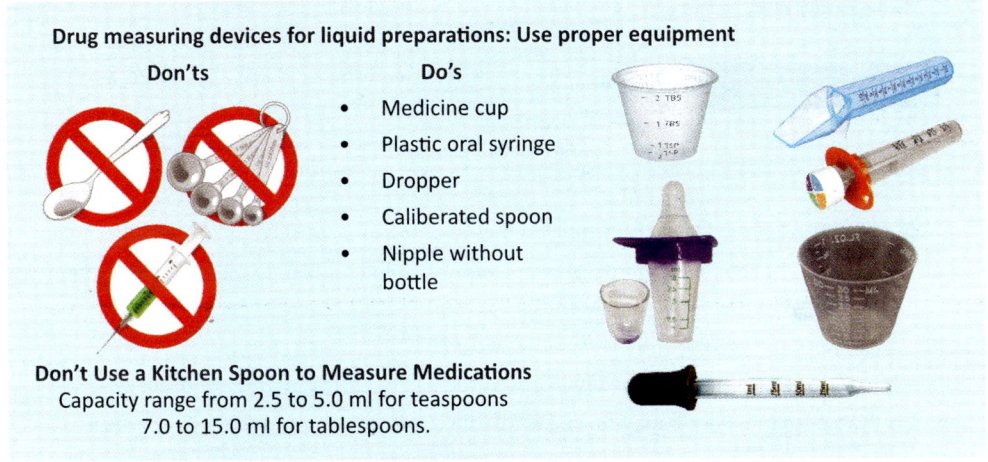

Drug measuring devices for liquid preparations: Use proper equipment

Don'ts	Do's
	• Medicine cup
	• Plastic oral syringe
	• Dropper
	• Caliberated spoon
	• Nipple without bottle

Don't Use a Kitchen Spoon to Measure Medications
Capacity range from 2.5 to 5.0 ml for teaspoons
7.0 to 15.0 ml for tablespoons.

5. Parents should be advised not to add any medicines to the infant's feed as

    i.   Drug may interact with the milk or other liquid in it.

    ii. Ingested dosage may be reduced, if the child does not drink all the contents.

6. It is particularly important to state the strengths of capsules or tablets/Syrups/kid tabs.

7. Many children may prefer a solid dose form. Parents may help in choosing the formulation.

8. Avoid painful intramuscular injections, whenever, possible.

9. Parents must be warned to keep all medicines out of reach of children.

10. Doses are generally based on body-weight (in kilograms) or the following age ranges:

    i.   first month (neonate)   ii. up to 1 year (infant)

    iii. 1-5 years   iv. 6-12 years

11. Children- Dose may be calculated from adult doses by using age, bodyweight, or body-surface area, or by a combination of these factors.

12. Young children may require a higher dose/kg than adults because of their higher metabolic rates.

13. Calculation by bodyweight in the obese child may result in much higher doses being administered than necessary; dose should be calculated from an ideal weight related to height and age. May utilize App available for calculating dose per kg.

14. Dose can be calculated using body-surface area (BSA)

    a.   The average body surface area of a 70-kilogram human is about 1.8 m^2.

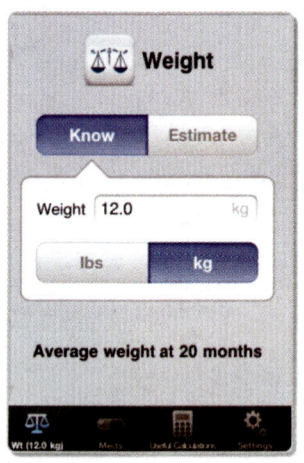

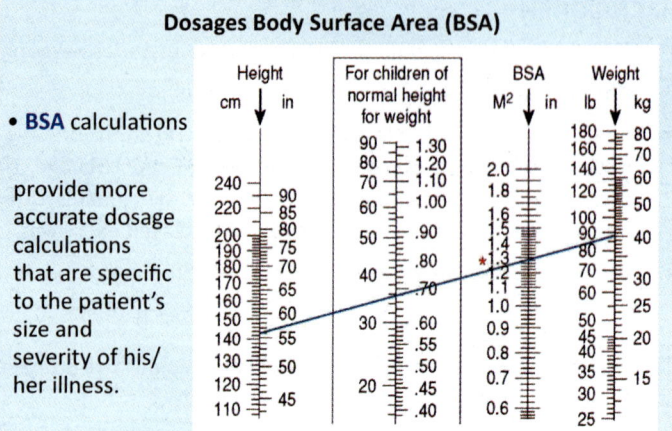

Dosages Body Surface Area (BSA)

• **BSA** calculations provide more accurate dosage calculations that are specific to the patient's size and severity of his/her illness.

$$\text{Approximate dose for patient} = \frac{\text{surface area of patient (m}^2)}{1.8} \times \text{adult dose}$$

15. Reporting of Adverse Drug reactions (ADRs) in children strongly encouraged because:

   i.   The action of the drug and its pharmacokinetics in children (especially in the very young) may be different from that in adults

   ii.   Drugs are not extensively tested in children

   iii. Many drugs are not specifically licensed for use in children and are used 'off-label'

   iv.   Suitable formulations may not be available to allow precise dosing in children

   v.   The nature and course of illnesses and adverse drug reactions may differ between adults and children.

B. ELDERLY

1. Obtain detailed drug history especially with reference to over-the-counter medication being taken by patient and if any of these fall under STOPP criteria[8].

2. Start with smaller dose & gradually increase

3. Keep the dosage schedule simple with minimum number of pills. Use dose boxes to improve adherence.

4. Review and check dosage modification, if any

5. Explain clearly and involve family members and friends for help.

6. Monitor therapeutic level for drugs with narrow therapeutic range (digoxin, lithium, phenytoin, etc.)

7. Consider cost of a medicine as limited economic resources may hamper procurement and consequently the compliance of medication

8. Monitor for side effects.

Review medications

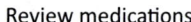

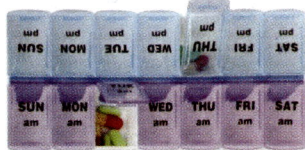

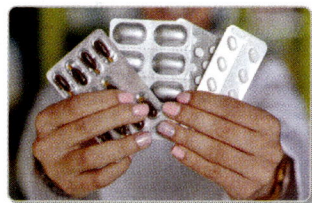

---

8 STOPP is the screening tool of older people's prescriptions as some drugs are potentially inappropriate for elderly patients and START is the screening tool to alert to right treatment (START) criteria.

C. PREGNANCY AND LACTATION

1. Some medications are harmful when taken during pregnancy, but others are unlikely to cause harm.

2. Only half of all pregnancies are planned.

3. Many women need medications for pregnancy induced conditions (e.g. morning sickness), chronic conditions (e.g. epilepsy), intercurrent conditions (allergies), etc.

4. Women working with chemicals, exposed to radiation and use illicit drugs - during embryogenesis may adversely affect foetal development

5. Effect of toxic drugs are:
   a. Malformation
   b. Growth retardation
   c. Foetal death
   d. Functional defects in newborn
   e. Premature birth

But use of drugs in pregnancy is not always wrong

1. High fever is harmful for the foetus in the first months. Use of paracetamol is better than no treatment.

2. Diabetes during pregnancy needs intensive therapy with insulin.

3. Folic acid protects against spina bifida.

4. Anti-epileptics are teratogenic. But an epileptic insult may provoke harmful anoxia for the foetus.

5. The pre-implantation period (day 1- 7) - damage of fertilized oocyte may lead to death or complete recovery.

6. The first trimester (day 8 – end of month 2) is the most important period for teratogenicity- is period of formation of organs.

7. 3rd – 9th month - Less risk for malformations except for urogenital tract, CNS.

8. More functional effects i.e. caused by drugs for example include
   o Aminoglycosides nephrotoxicity & ototoxicity
   o Salicylates increased risk of bleeding

Risk Classification

1. No drug is proven free from teratogenic effects, however some drugs have low risk whereas have higher risk.

2. Risk classification of FDA as A, B, C, D, X Drug risks to the foetus runs from: Category A (safest) → Category X (known danger – DO NOT USE)

3. May consult online resources such as FDA or other authentic website www.safefetus.com; www.perinatology.com/exposures/druglist.htm

Drug use in lactation

1. The amount of drug ingested by breastfeeding is difficult to assess, therefore, use the lowest possible dose.

2. Observe child closely

3. Observe time of drug intake versus breast feeding

4. Avoid drugs like
   i. Aminoglycosides
   ii. Thyrostatics
   iii. Chloramphenicol
   iv. Tetracyclines
   v. Immunosuppressants
   vi. Cytostatics

D. PSYCHIATRY DISORDERS

Medicines are used in case of a psychiatric illness or for psychiatric symptoms associated with physical illness or adverse effects of the medicines.

1. Medications often needed to be taken for long period, sometimes many years.
2. Assess compliance regularly as often medicines need to be taken even after the target symptoms have remitted – as maintenance or for prophylaxis.
3. Some medications like lithium, valproate may need regular blood level monitoring. Liver and renal function and blood counts required in other cases such as clozapine.
4. Patient should maintain regular contact with the psychiatrist.

V. DISPENSING OF SCHEDULE H1 DRUGS

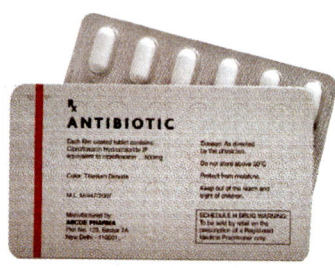

While most drugs are prescription only i.e., Schedule H in India, the government had included a new provision, Schedule H1 to the Drugs and Cosmetics Act in 2013 to check the indiscriminate use of some medicines over-the-counter as self medication of these medicines can be harmful. As many as 46 drugs were placed under this restricted category which mainly comprises third and fourth generation antibiotics, anti-TB and some other drugs. Hydroxychloroquine has been recently added to this list. See box below for the drugs included in Schedule H1.

The packaging of these drugs have mandatory warning printed on them in a box with a red border on the label and are to be sold by pharmacist on production of a valid prescription only.

A separate register should be maintained for these 47 drugs where the name of the patient and the details of the doctor who prescribed the drugs should be noted. This register should be kept for three years and be open for inspection by the regulatory authority.

Schedule H1					
1.	Alprazolam	17.	Ceftriaxone	33.	Meropenem
2.	Balofloxacin	18.	Chlordiazepoxide	34.	Midazolam
3.	Buprenorphine	19.	Clofazimine	35.	Moxifloxacin
4.	Capreomycin	20.	Codeine	36.	Nitrazepam
5.	Cefdinir	21.	Cycloserine	37.	Pentazocine
6.	Cefditoren	22.	Diazepam	38.	Prulifloxacin
7.	Cefepime	23.	Diphenoxylate	39.	Pyrazinamide
8.	Cefetamet	24.	Doripenem	40.	Rifabutin
9.	Cefexime	25.	Ertapenem	41.	Rifampicin
10.	Cefoperazone	26.	Ethambutol HCl	42.	Sodium Para-aminosalicylate
11.	Cefotaxime	27.	Ethinamide	43.	Sparfloxacin
12.	Cefpirome	28.	Feropenem	44.	Thiacetazone
13.	Cefpodoxime	29.	Gemifloxacin	45.	Tramadol
14.	Ceftazidime	30.	Imipenem	46.	Zolpidem
15.	Ceftibuten	31.	Isoniazid	47.	Hydroxychloroquine
16.	Ceftizoxime	32.	Levofloxacin		

VI. NARCOTIC AND PSYCHOTROPIC DRUGS (NDP)

To exercise control on the use of NDPS such as opium derivatives, morphine and pethidine with abuse potential Narcotics and Psychotropic Substances Act, 1985 was passed and such substances are entered in Schedule "X" of Drugs and Cosmetic Act, 1940. For details also see section on handling of NDPS. Amendment in 2014 included a notified list of Essential Narcotic Drugs (ENDs) for medical and scientific use for regulation & control under Drugs & Cosmetics Act to improve access to these medicines. The list included morphine, methadone, codeine, hydrocodone, oxycodone and its salts and fentanyl. The ENDs can be stocked by 'Recongnized Medical Institution' (RMIs) authorized by the State Drugs Controller. The authorization is for 3 years and is renewable. Government hospitals are deemed RMIs provided mandated requirements as below are followed:

1. These medicines should be procured from authorized dealers/suppliers only.

2. The ENDs should be prescribed as per Rules and dispensed only to select patients registered with the RMI and record of the dispensing maintained in a format as prescribed under the Rules (Form No. 3E under rule 52H(3)] . This record should be retained for two years from the date of last entry.

3. This record shall be maintained on day-to-day basis and entries should be made for each day before the close of the day for each essential narcotic drug separately in a register with pages serially numbered. Separate record should be maintained for each essential narcotic drug. This record should be retained for two years from the date of last entry. This record should be produced before the concerned authorized officers on inspection/investigation.

4. The ENDs stock with the RMI should not be transferred, loaned or sold to other institutions except with the written permission of the State Drug Controller.

A. DISPENSING ESSENTIAL NARCOTIC DRUGS (ENDs)

1. To dispense ENDs, a pharmacist must know the requirements for a valid prescription which are described below in this section.

2. While maintaining stock of these drugs they should be kept under lock and key and must be accurately received and issued. A separate register should be maintained to record them and a controlled procedure is used to issue or receive these drugs.

3. Medical Superintendent is overall responsible for handling of ENDs. Chief pharmacist procures stores and is responsible for proper dispensing of drugs within the hospital.

4. A prescription must be written in ink or indelible pencil or typewritten and must be manually signed by the practitioner on the date when issued.

5. Only designated registered medical practitioners (RMPs) within appropriate clinic system are authorized to write prescriptions for drugs that fall under their area of expertise. In case of individual RMPs the prescription can be prescribed only by those approved Practitioners who are either registered with Collector of Excise on this behalf and have obtained Registration Certificate in form DD-8 or holding a License in Form DD-5. A registered dentist should give a prescription only for the purpose of dental treatment and shall make if 'for local dental treatment only'. Non-psychiatric consultants may only prescribe psychotropic drugs, if the use of such drugs falls under their area of specialization or patient management. Fellows and residents may write prescriptions for regular drugs when working with consultants in their clinics. However, a consultant must countersign prescriptions for ENDs. The designated RMP is responsible for ensuring the prescription conforms to all requirements of the law and regulations, both federal and state.

6. The designated RMP should write on official prescription form. The prescription for a ENDs should rewritten and should not be repeated as 'continue same treatment'.

7. There should be no strikeover, erasures or mispellings of the drug name, strength or quantity.

8. A registered pharmacy may process electronic prescriptions for ENDs only if all of the applicable requirements are met.

9. A complete prescription for ENDs must include the following information:

   i. Patient's full name, address and if appropriate date of birth, if any other family members shares the same name.

   ii. Address

   iii. Date

   iv. Name and strength of the drug in Capitals and dosage form, daily dose and duration

   v. Total quantity of drug to be supplied

   vi. Full name, qualification and signature of the Approved Practitioner

   vii. Name of the Licensed Chemist who dispensed the prescription and date

10. The complete ENDs prescription must be written on a hospital prescription form by registered medical practitioner and then it is signed and sent to the hospital pharmacy. Abbreviation like p.r.n (Pro Re Nata) or S.O.S. (Si Opus Sit) must be discouraged for such drugs.

    The completed form along with the empty containers and nurses inventory sheet is sent to the pharmacy for dispensing. The prescription signed by Registered Medical Practitioner will also permit the patient to purchase drug from outside pharmacy.

11. The pharmacist should check the prescription for completeness and dispense the drugs as a unit-dose.

12. All prescriptions must be dated at the time of writing and are valid for filling in the pharmacy for example:

    i. Within 24 hours, if written in emergency room (ER prescriptions for ENDs are dispensed for 3 days only).

    ii. Seven days, if generated from clinics (OPD) prescriptions.

13. The pharmacist in-charge will not dispense the prescription if:

    i. The prescription is not complete.

    ii. The patient received the medication and still has amount left for another 7 days.

    iii. Potential drug-drug interaction.

    iv. Any suspicion of fraud (strikeover, erasure) in the prescription and the patient must be informed.

    v Misspellings of the drug name, strength or quantity.

14. After dispensing the prescription, put a "DISPENSED" stamp. DO NOT dispense more then the prescribed quantity. While preparing the bill, write the complete name & address of the doctor, and the patient with the exact quantity of medicines dispensed, batch no -DO NOT HOME deliver and DO NOT accept telephonic order.

    i. Never SUBSTITUTE such medicines. Contact the doctor in case of unavailability or any other problem.

ii. In case of any doubts, like huge quantity prescribed or a suspicious character with a bogus prescription, immediately contact and confirm with the doctor/ prescriber, OR POLITELY REFUSE to dispense the prescription.

15. Provide complete information to the patient about the prescribed drug dispensed including cautions, warnings and clear direction for use.

16. Under the current regulation, the pharmacist is not permitted either to refill or substitute a generically equivalent narcotic drug unless instructed by the physician.

17. Closely monitor repeat prescriptions.

18. The name and address of each patient for whom END was prescribed is entered in the register along with the quantity disbursed. Record of every patient to whom END was dispensed should be maintained in the format of Form 3E.

Known risks

- Unauthorised person prescribing or transcribing of a narcotic prescription
- Supply of a narcotic prescribed by an unauthorised person
- Supply of a narcotic against a prescription that does not meet the legal and local requirements
- Potential for a substance misuse patient to access prescriptions from two sources for the same period.

B. Preparation of ENDs against a prescription prior to administration and recording of details

1. Validation of the prescription

It must not be assumed that the person prescribing the ENDs is authorized to do so. Care must be taken by staff to ensure as far as reasonably possible that the prescription is valid. If in doubt of the validity of the signature, steps must be taken in order to verify their authority to prescribe. For details see section on Handling of Narcotics and Psychotropic Substances.

2. Preparation and administration of the dose against the prescription

The procedure for administration of a ENDs is the same as for other medicines. In addition:

i. The person administering must be aware of the following characteristics of the medicine and formulation: usual starting dose, frequency of administration, standard dosing increments, symptoms of overdose and common side effects.

ii. When a dose increase is prescribed, the calculated dose should be checked to ensure that it is safe for the patient, not normally more than 50% higher than the previous dose.

iii. Confirm with the prescriber any dose that appears to be unusual. In addition, all ENDs except temazepam, morphine liquid preparations of 10mg in 5ml or less must be checked and administered by two people, one of whom must be a Registered Nurse or a Registered medical practitioner. The second person (witness) should preferably be any of these or a pharmacist. The witness should observe the whole procedure including the preparation and the administration. Both staff must have seen a valid prescription for the ENDs and any wastage for the patient prior to administration.

iv. Liquid ENDs can often be marginally out due to small but repeated errors in the measuring process, may cause problems on reconciliation. This can be reduced by using the smallest measuring device possible e.g., oral syringes for lower doses.

v.   Staff administering ENDs must be competent to recognize and treat any patient deterioration and/or any known adverse effect that required immediate life support intervention, such as anaphylaxis, cardiovascular collapse, respiratory depression.

vi.   Closely supervise substance misuse by patients of their doses to ensure that they have actually taken the medication.

vii. Exercise extra scrutiny and staff should be aware of the consequences of incomplete administration especially substance misusers and patients in psychiatric wards.

viii. Record details of the administration in the ward ENDs Record Book, together with a full signature of both the witness and the person who administered the drug.

ix.   The Record Book must be completed immediately following the administration of the ENDs.

x.   If the ENDs is wasted or only partially used, it should be destroyed in the presence of the witness and a record made in the ENDs Register which is prepared as per Form 3H and record of day-to-day every transaction is made in the format of Form 3D duly verified by the doctor-in-charge at the end of the daily entry. A record must also be made in the ENDs Record Book to that effect stating the amount administered and the amount wasted, together with signatures of the two people concerned.

> **Known risks**
> - Administration of invalid prescription to a patient
> - Unauthorised staff completing the preparation and administration processes.
> - Inaccurate doses prepared or administered to patients
> - Incomplete records of administered or missed doses and dose incidents resulting in duplication or inappropriate administration
> - Inaccurate completion or failure to complete the ENDs register
> - Inadequate training/competence of staff to deliver each aspect of the SOP.

C.   DELIVERY TO INPATIENTS/WARDS/FLOORS

1. All parts of the transportation system should protect the medication from pilferage and breakage.

2. Special procedures for delivery of ENDs should be established to ensure that the drugs are delivered promptly, intact and placed in proper storage areas.

3. The delivery of narcotic drugs from the pharmacy to the wards and nursing stations must be carried out through some reliable persons.

4. Medication should be delivered to the ward from the pharmacy with the least amount of delay.

5. After the dispensing of narcotics by the pharmacy, nurses resume the responsibility for administration, control and auditing of the inventory. Nurses on duty count physically narcotics on each nursing station to check the records.

6. While administering a dose, if patient refuses or doctor cancels any dose, it is the duty of the nurse to destroy the drug into sink and record "Refused by patient" or "order cancelled by doctor". Nurses should always maintain a proper record in case of wastage/destruction/contamination.

7. The unused drugs, due to discontinuation as a result of discharge or expiration of the patient, must be returned to the pharmacist in-charge.

8. On discharge, the patient is issued a new prescription to be dispensed only to the Head Nurse, who will forward the medication to the patient.

Recording

1. ENDs Log Book should be maintained for daily recording.

2. In the ENDs log book, the pharmacist should give the END forms each a serial number, and record all the required information in the book.

3. Record of the day-to-day entries is maintained. A monthly statistics of the consumed drugs is prepared by the pharmacist and sent to the appropriate authorities.

4. The inventory must check every 3 months by a committee formed by the Head of the hospital, one of the members from Inventory control management in hospital.

Inspection

1. The Pharmacist in-charge should monthly check the expiration date of the ENDs in the pharmacy.

2. The Nurse-in-charge should check the expiration date of the ENDs in their respective wards regularly.

3. If the drug is nearly expired and is not moving in a specific ward, it should be returned to the pharmacy by the Nurse-in-charge 3 month before the expiration date, and the Pharmacy will distribute it to those wards in which it may be used before it expires.

D. PHARMACIST IN-CHARGE OF ESSENTIAL NARCOTIC DRUGS (ENDS) RESPONSIBILITIES

1. Although support staff (pharmacists and nurses) may manage the day-to-day entries, the medical officer in-charge has primary responsibility of the stock and dispensing ENDs.

2. Keep all ENDs in a locked cabinet under his/her own direct supervision and control.

3. Must check validity of the prescription and identity of the patient before dispensing.

4. Consult the prescribing doctor if there is any doubt about the prescription.

5. Only dispense ENDs if the prescription provided by the physician is complete and valid. Dispensing part of a prescription is not permitted.

6. Properly label and mark containers to avoid undue intermixing that may cause harm to the patient. .

7. Prepare & Signs quarterly reports to appropriate authorities as custodian.

8. Maintains adequate stock of all ENDs to meet user unit's requirements. . The total quantity possessed by the RMI at any one time, should not exceed the submitted estimate (or revised estimate if any). This quantity may be ordered repeatedly during the year, if the need for ENDs scales up during the year. If the requirement for ENDs has increased during the course of the year, the officer in-charge of the RMI can submit the revised estimate for the same year by the 31st August. A brief justification for the same should be provided while filing the annual return in Form 3I.

File annual return to the Controller of drugs, for the calendar year on or before 31st of March of the subsequent year in the format of Form 3I.

9. Do not allow any unauthorized person (hospital staff, patients, visitors, etc.) inside the ENDs room or give keys of these controlled drugs receptacle.

10. Allow only pharmacy staff, operation theatre and anaesthesia department technicians, and nursing staff who are assigned to receive and replace these medications through secure window.

11. Maintain clear, legible and accurate perpetual inventory records of all ENDs under his/ her custody with no crossing-out erasures or overwriting.

12. Issue/replenish ENDs upon receipt of one of the following, properly prepared and signed, documents:

    i. Essential Narcotic drugs prescriptions.

    ii. Reports of broken or lost ampoules, (replenishment of what has been lost or wasted)

    iii. Essential Narcotic Drug prescription forms, (for discharged patients, out-patients).

13. Revise the above listed issue documents for accuracy and to ensure that they are properly completed, without crossing-out, erasures or over-writing, before dispensing/replenishing the drug.

14. Prepare documents for the destruction of empty ampoules/vial at the end of the month.

15. Prepare & ensures that original signed stock level lists for user units maintained in the pharmacy are up-to-date and accurate.

16. Take immediate action to ensure that any change(s) is/are reflected on the stock level list, as follows:

    i. Change the list, item which is being added.

    ii. Initials with date.

    iii. Revise and update the list as required.

17. Keep the following permanent, separate (ENDs) files in good order: Issue documents file, including:

    i. Report loss or waste;

    ii. Required documents for ENDs purchasing and receiving;

    iii. Required documents related to the destruction of empty ampoules and the expired ENDs;

    iv. Any memo sent by Ministry of Health (MOH) to the hospital related to Narcotic & Psychotropic drugs.

VII. CONDITIONS OF PHARMACY PREMISES AND STORAGE OF MEDICINES IN PHARMACY

A. RESPONSIBILITIES OF THE PHARMACIST

1. Pharmacy owners must recognize and facilitate compliance with their relevant legal obligations.

2. All registered pharmacists have an obligation to ensure the pharmacy is operated in accordance with all legislation and guidance, promoting the highest professional standards in the delivery of pharmacy care, treatment and service.

3. Must ensure that the premises and facilities are fit for purpose for the provision of pharmacy services and are well maintained, facilitating a safe and effective working environment and reflecting the professional nature of a healthcare facility.

4. The pharmacy owner should provide and maintain such staff, premises, equipment and procedures for the storage, preparation, dispensing, compounding, sale and supply of medicinal products as per legal requirements.

5. The pharmacist must be able to effectively control all medicinal products and confidential records within the pharmacy, including all areas accessible to employees, and no unauthorized access must be permitted.

B. SIZE, LAYOUT AND ORGANISATION OF PHARMACY

1. The dispensary size and layout must facilitate an uninterrupted, safe and efficient work-flow and permit effective and direct supervision by the pharmacist of, and effective communication between, all staff involved in the preparing, compounding or dispensing of medicinal products.

2. The dispensary should be organised to keep distractions to a minimum and provide for the safe delivery of patient care.

3. Sufficient space must be available for the safe and effective storage of all dispensary medicines and medicines should be stored at an accessible shelf height i.e., pharmacy staff should not have to reach excessively to access them.

4. A designated, adequate and secure space must be provided in the dispensary for the storage of prescription medicines and secure storage for narcotic drugs.

5. The dispensary should be well-lit and sufficiently ventilated and must be maintained hygienically and be free from all sources of contamination.

6. The dispensary must have arrangements for the proper storage and disposal of all types of waste materials.

7. Sufficient storage space should be allocated to allow the orderly management of stock and effective stock rotation.

8. All fixtures and fittings within the dispensary must be fully finished to a high standard and in good condition, suitable and adequate for the purpose for which they were intended. Appropriate shelving and fixtures must be in place so that no medicinal products are stored on the floor, on stairs, in passageways or in toilets.

9. All storage areas and facilities within the registered premises, including fixtures and fittings, walls, ceiling and paintwork must be in keeping with that expected from a health care facility and maintained to a high standard. Storage areas should be self-contained.

10. Control and supervision must be demonstrable with appropriate security and stock control policies and procedures in place.

11. Adequate staff facilities should be available, including a separate area for staff to prepare and eat food. Eating must not be permitted in the dispensing area.

12. Adequate heating and lighting should be provided in all employee areas.

13. Entry to all staff areas and facilities, including stock rooms, toilet facilities, communal areas and administration offices must be controlled and restricted.

14. Provision should be made for toilet and hand-washing facilities for staff, with both hot and cold water.

15. The toilet area should not open directly into the dispensary and must not be used for storage. Hand washing posters should be displayed in the toilet area.

C. POLICIES AND PROCEDURES

1. Pharmacists should ensure that there are written policies and procedures in place for all aspects of premises requirements outlined in these guidelines and for any pharmacy-specific methods of premises maintenance.

2. Cleaning and maintenance procedures should be developed and maintained for all areas of the premises.

3. There should be procedures in place which outline the processes involved in maintaining effective security, including security assessments, on-going security audits and appropriate training of personnel.

4. Every pharmacy should have documented procedures and policies in place to facilitate compliance with all relevant Building and Fire Regulations as well as Health and Safety legislation.

D. STORAGE OF MEDICINES IN PHARMACY

1. Medicines and chemicals must normally be stored in the manufacturer's original containers. Do not remove medicines from original packing. If, in exceptional cases and with due consideration of the nature of the product concerned, the contents need to be transferred to other containers, care must be taken to avoid contamination and all relevant information must be marked clearly on the new container.

2. All materials must be stored under suitable conditions, appropriate to the nature and stability of the material concerned. Particular attention must be paid to protection from contamination, sunlight, atmospheric moisture and adverse temperatures.

3. A pharmacist must exercise his/her knowledge of stability of materials to segregate for disposal and destroy any substances which have deteriorated as per procedure laid down or which have been in stock for unduly long periods, or which have reached their expiry dates.

4. Ensure adequate space for storage of medicines
   i. Label facing forward
   ii. Agents for external use should never be stored with oral medications
   iii. Separate by route of administration
   iv. Mark and/or isolate high-alert drugs
   v. Separate sound-alike/ look-alike drugs

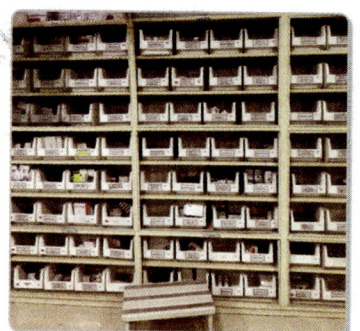 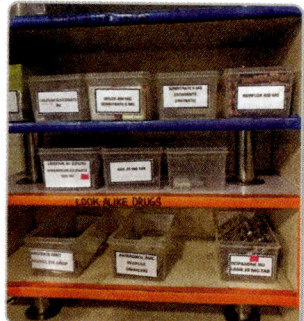

For details see section on Medical Stores Management

E. EXPIRY DATES—MANAGEMENT

1. The pharmacist must ensure that the product dispensed remain in-dated for the duration of treatment.

2. Particular care should be taken with prescriptions for several months treatment. Ideally prescriptions should be for a maximum of 28 days' treatment or as per hospital policy but, where a quantity covering a longer period is dispensed, the pharmacist must ensure that the product will still be in-date at the end of that period.

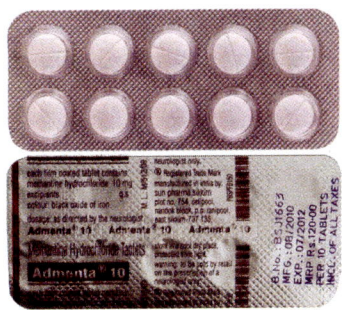

3. If the date on the label has a specific month, day, and year, the medicine/vaccine can be used through the end of that day (e.g. 20/05/2010 – use through 20/05/2015). If the expiration date on the label is a month and year, the medicine/vaccine can be used through the last day of that month (e.g. 12/2015 – use through 12/31/2015). For details see section on Preventing Expiry in Medical Stores.

F. PERSONAL HYGIENE

1. High standards of personal cleanliness must be observed in dispensing.

2. Direct contact between the dispensed product and the operator's hands must be avoided.

3. Cuts or abrasions must be covered with a suitable occlusive dressing. A person with an open lesion or readily transmittable infection must report to the pharmacist who will decide whether they may be engaged in the dispensing process.

4. No personnel may smoke or prepare or consume food in any area where medicines are dispensed, sold or supplied.

G. REUSE/RETURNED MEDICATIONS

A pharmacist must use his/her professional knowledge in relation to reuse of medicines as follows:

1. Medicines brought in by patients:
   i. All such medicines are the patients' own property.
   ii. Under no circumstances may they be considered for reuse by anyone else.

2. Medicines returned from a hospital ward:
   i. All expired medicines must be destroyed as per hospital policy;
   ii. Owing to the inherent danger, drugs having different lot numbers and expiry dates should not be combined.

3. Medications dispensed for administration, but not used, should be returned to the pharmacy. Only blister packs may be considered for re-use provided that the pharmacist is confident that the correct storage conditions have been adhered to; and procedures for returning drugs to stock should be instituted. These should include the following considerations:
   i. Integrity of returned drug package
   ii. Proper storage of the drug on the nursing care station

4. The following types of medication should be discarded:

    i. Any opened topical medications (including ophthalmic, ear and nasal medications)

    ii. Opened multi-dose and single dose vials

    iii. Any medication handled by the patient

    iv. Any medications returned by ambulatory patients

    v. Improperly stored medications

    vi. Any open or used IV admixtures

    vii. Any opened liquid medications

5. The continued use of patients' own medicines while in hospital may be necessary in special circumstances. Appropriate safeguards are required and any system for handling such medicines must be in accordance with current Good Pharmacy Practice.

VIII. RECALLS

A drug recall is a voluntary action taken by a manufacturer/hospital to remove a defective drug product from the market/hospital that violate requirements and that may represent a health hazard to the consumer/user.

The withdrawal/recall of a particular batch or batches of a product from the market/hospital may be occasioned by the following:

- Serious reports of adverse drug reactions not included in the package insert
- Unexpected frequency of adverse reaction stated in the package inserts
- Incorrect labelling of a product
- Incorrect formulation of a product
- Found to be defective on quality assurance

A. LEVEL OF RECALL

1. Level of recall refers to the part of the distribution chain to which the recall is extended, (wholesale, retail, pharmacy, medical user, etc.) It is necessary to assign/indicate the relative degree of health hazard presented by the product being recalled, namely:

2. The following classification criterion is recommended:

    Class I is for defective/dangerous/potentially life-threatening medicines that predictably or probably could result into serious health risk/adverse events or even death.

    Class II is for medicines that possibly could cause temporary or medically reversible adverse health problem or mistreatment.

    Class III is for medicines that is defective and is unlikely to cause any adverse health reaction or which do not comply with the requirements of the Drugs & Cosmetics Act, in terms of the requirements of printed packaging material, product specification, labelling, etc.

B. TYPES OF RECALL

1. A Type A recall is designed to reach all suppliers of medicines (all distribution points) i.e. wholesalers throughout the country, directors of hospital services (private as well as state hospitals), retail outlets, doctors, nurses, pharmacists, authorised prescribers and dispensers and individual customers or patients through media release (radio, television, regional and

national press). Recall letter is sent to all distribution points plus media release.

2. A Type B recall is designed to reach wholesalers throughout the country, directors of hospital services (private as well as state hospitals), retail outlets, doctors, nurses, pharmacists, authorised prescribers and dispensers. Recall letter is sent to all distribution points.

3. A Type C recall is designed to reach wholesale level and other distribution points (e.g. pharmacies, doctors, hospitals). This can be achieved by means of representatives calling on wholesalers and/or retail outlets. If it is known where the product in question had been distributed to, specific telephone calls or recalls letters to arrange for the return of the product could be made. Specific telephone calls, recall letters to/representatives calling at distribution points if known where the medicines have been distributed.

C. BASIC INFORMATION REQUIRED FOR RECALL

1. Name, strength, pack size, batch/lot number and any means of identification of the recalled product; Total quantity of the product being recalled originally in possession of the company

2. The date distribution of the product began

3. The total quantity of the product being recalled that had been distributed up to the time of the recall should be indicated.

4. Area of distribution of the product and, if exported, the country to where it was exported.

5. List of customers to whom product was issued

6. The quantity of the recalled product still in their possession

7. The reason for initiating the recall; nature of defect

8. Suggested action to be taken and its urgency

9. Indication of the health risk together with reasons

D. ROLE OF PHARMACISTS DURING A RECALL

1. During a recall, the primary role of the Pharmacy is to closely monitor the effectiveness of the companies'/hospitals recall actions.

2. A pharmacist must comply immediately with any warning about or recall of defective medicines.

3. Every institutional pharmacy should have a recall policy to ensure that the defective medicine will be obtained from the wards and satellite pharmacies.

4. A pharmacist should actively participate in any arrangements made for warning the profession of problems associated with medicines, and should inform appropriate bodies of hazards which come to their attention.

5. A recall is terminated when the Pharmacy and the recalling company are in agreement that the non-compliant product has been removed and proper disposal or correction has been made.

Sometimes error may occur in the process of ordering, transcribing, dispensing, administering and monitoring a medication. A medication error may or may not result in an actual or potential adverse drug event. Top Error Categories include surgical complications, wrong side surgery, medication errors and blood Transfusion errors.

I. DEFINITIONS:

Sentinel Event: An occurrence unplanned, not scheduled or anticipated, resulting in death, serious harm, or the risk for physical or psychological harm.

Near miss: A near miss (a.k.a. close call) is an unplanned event that did not result in injury to the patient. Only a fortunate break in the chain of events prevented injury. The immediate challenge is to identify interventions that can reduce near miss errors until the more expensive technological solutions can be implemented. Error is an opportunity to learn and correct system failures before harm reaches the patient.

Medication Error: Any preventable event that may cause or lead to inappropriate medication use or patient harm while the medication is in the control of the health care professional, patient or consumer. A major medication error is one which results in either permanent harm or transfer to the ICU.

DISPENSING ERRORS

A dispensing error is a discrepancy between a prescription and the medicine that the pharmacy delivers to the patient or distributes to the ward on the basis of this prescription indent, including the dispensing of a medicine with inferior pharmaceutical or informational quality.

II. CASE STUDIES

1. A 60 years old female patient was prescribed Syr. Eptoin (Phenytoin) 15 ml, three times a day after craniotomy. Since Syr. Eptoin was not available in pharmacy, it was substituted by another brand Dilantin. Eptoin contains (30 mg/5 ml of Phenytoin) while Syr. Dilantin contains (125 mg/5 ml of Phenytoin). The patient received 1025 mg of phenytoin instead of 270 mg for 5 days, this resulted in abnormal CT changes and patient remained drowsy for 7 days.

2. An elderly man was admitted to intensive care with hyperkalaemia as a result of a dispensing error. The pharmacist had mixed up the prescriptions. As a result, this man received another person's medications, including a potassium supplement. Unfortunately, the patient had a history of renal failure and required many months of haemodialysis as a result.

3. An elderly lady experienced a prolonged period of hospitalization for renal failure as a result

of a dispensing error. Although she was prescribed Methotrexate weekly, the pharmacist inadvertently dispensed a daily dose to her.

4. Fentanyl was prescribed at the incorrect concentration (50 mg/ml). Fentanyl (0.05 mg/ml) was dispensed without asking for concentration confirmation from the prescriber.

5. Morphine (10 mg) was prescribed without the dosage form. An injectable solution was dispensed when tablet was also available at a 10 mg concentration.

6. For a patient suffering from epilepsy the doctor ordered Tab. Valproic acid CR 500mg in the prescription but the pharmacist dispensed Valproic acid 500 mg. Patient continued to have seizure and doctor increased the dose to 800 mg/day. Then on third visit after one month dose was further increased to 1000 mg/day as seizures were not controlled. On review of medications being taken by the patient it was discovered that though CR preparation was prescribed but patient had been receiving plain preparation only.

7. Patient suffering from depression was prescribed Imipramine 25 mg HS for 3 days then 50 mg HS for next 3 days, then 75 mg at night for one month and to be continued for 3 month. Patient initially responded but later depressive symptoms appeared again. On enquiring it was observed that patient was taking 25 mg tablet at bedtime daily.

8. Dispensing errors include dispensing the incorrect drug, dose, dosage form, wrong quantity or inappropriate, incorrect or inadequate labeling. Also, confusing or inadequate directions for use, incorrect or inappropriate preparation, packaging or storage of medication prior to dispensing are considered to be errors. Often brand substitution is being made by pharmacist without realizing the correctness of the dispensed drugs.

III. DISPENSING ERRORS: WHO IS AT MOST RISK

A. PATIENTS RECEIVING LOOK-ALIKE, SOUND-ALIKE (LASA) DRUGS

1. Many drug names look or sound like other drug names. Dispensing errors are common due to lookalike, sound alike (LASA) and spell alike drugs and is a concern world wide. With tens of thousands of drugs currently on the market, the potential for error due to confusing drug names is significant. This includes nonproprietary names and proprietary (brand or trade marked) names.

2. Contributing to this confusion are illegible handwriting, incomplete knowledge of drug names, newly available products, similar packaging or labeling, similar clinical use, similar strengths, dosage forms, frequency of administration, and the failure of manufacturers and regulatory authorities to recognize the potential for error and to conduct rigorous risk assessments, both for nonproprietary and brand names, prior to approving new product names. Brand names are developed by the product's sponsor and often differ significantly between countries. Some medicines, although marketed under the same or similar-sounding brand names may contain different active ingredients in different countries. Furthermore, the same drug marketed by more than one company may have more than one brand name.

3. The increasing potential for LASA medication errors was recognized by the Accreditation Board and was incorporated into the National Patient Safety Goals that requires each accredited organization to identify a list of look-alike or sound-alike drugs used in the organization.

4. Some examples of name pairs that have caused confusion in several countries around the world are shown below:

Confusing medication names (sound similar or appear similar) may lead to potentially harmful medication errors contributing to adverse events.

Examples of similar names of different drugs and formulations and sound alike (LASA) drugs

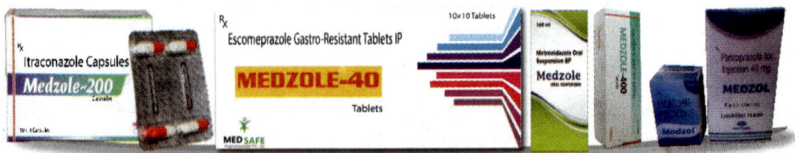

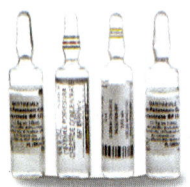 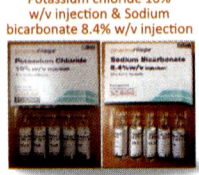 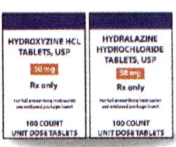 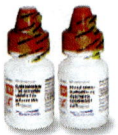 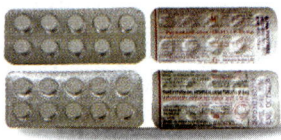

Examples of some confusing drug name pairs. Brand name followed by Nonproprietary name shown in bold):

PAM (**pralidoxime**) PAN (**pantaprazole**)

Avanza (**mirtazapine**) Avandia (**rosiglitazone**)

Losec (**omeprazole**) Lasix (**frusemide**)

Diamox (**acetazolamide**) Zimox (**amoxicillina triidrato**)

Dianben (**metformin**) Diovan (**valsartan**)

Ecazide (**captopril/hydrochlorothiazide**) Eskazine (**trifluoperazine**)

Lantus (**insulin glargine**) Lanvis (**toguanine**)

Daonil (**glibenclamide**) Diavol (**Antacid**)

Glynase (**glyburide**) Zinase (**Serratiopeptidase**)

Incidal (**cetirizine**) Inderal (**propranolol**)

..............Thousands more, some reported, most not

5. LASA drugs should be identified and updated in inpatient (IP) & outpatient (OP) Pharmacy frequently and information should be disseminated to all areas where drugs are used (wards/ Floors, ICUs, emergency, Operation theaters (OT's). See following section on Dispensing errors for details.

B. USE OF ABBREVIATIONS, SYMBOLS AND DOSE DESIGNATIONS

1. Abbreviations of drug names

The common abbreviation for "hydrochlorthiazide 50 mg' HCTZ was misread as "hydrocortisone 250 mg." In another case, an order for "AZT 100 mg" (a common abbreviation for the antiretroviral drug zidovudine) for a patient with AIDS, was misinterpreted as azathioprine, an immunosuppressant. The potential harm in giving azathioprine to a patient with AIDS is obvious.

Write full name of the drug.

2. Stemmed drug names

"Nitro' drip for nitroglycerine mistaken as sodium nitroprusside infusion; "Norflox" for norfloxacin mistaken as norflex (Orphenadrine); "IV Vanc" for vancomycin mistaken as INVANZ (Ertapenem).

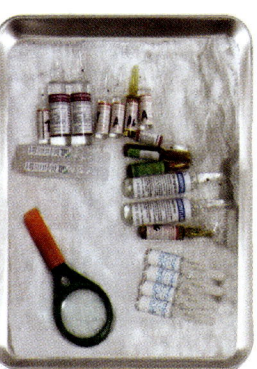

Write full name of the drug.

3. Space between drug and strength & Reading Small letters

No space between drug and strength may be misread. For example:

- Tegretol300 mg misread as Tagretol 1300 mg.
- Inderal40 mg misread as inderal 140 mg

Give space between drug and strength. Use lens to read small letters.

4. Dose strength abbreviations

The abbreviated form 'µg' is very easily misread as 'mg', a 1000-fold overdose.

Handwritten abbreviated form ('U') for 'Units' is very easily misread as '0 or 4'.

Always write out "Unit".

The strength of the drug should be stated in standard units using abbreviations that are consistent with the System Internationale (SI).

5. Medication errors from decimal

Avoid decimals whenever possible. Write 125 mcg" instead of 0.125 mg. Do not write naked or trailing decimal ('.5' or '1.0') as .5 mg can read as 5 mg and 0.1 mg be read as 1 mg.

"Lead don't trail", if unavoidable, a zero should be written in front of the decimal point (e.g. '0.5'). Never write -1.0mg it can be mis-read as 10 mg.

6. Misreading Letters and Numbers

Abbreviation - mg. or ml. with a period following the abbreviation can be misread as the number if written poorly.

Mixups: between "l" and the number "1; "O" &"0,"; "Z" & "2,"; "1" & "7" are also common.

Some more examples of error-prone abbreviation contributing to potential and actual errors, submitted to the Institute For Safe Medication Practices Medication Errors Reporting Programme are:

Error prone abbreviations, symbols and dose designations					
Abbreviation	Intended meaning	Misinterpretation	Abbreviation	Intended meaning	Misinterpretation
@	at	2	1.0ml	1ml	10ml
+	Plus/and	4	.5mg	0.5mg	5mg
µg	microgram	mg or ng	100000 units	1,00,000	10,000/1,000,000
IJ	injection	IV	U or u	Unit	0/4
IU	International units	IV	X3d	For 3 days	3 doses
OD	Once daily	Right eye	q1d	daily	4 times daily
10 mg		1 if written poorly	qhs	Nightly at bed time	Qhr or every hour

7. Route of Administration

A prescriber wrote a prescription intending the patient to receive hypertonic saline via a nebulizer. However, the prescriber used the ambiguous abbreviation "NMT" to signify the route. The pharmacist was accustomed to prescribers using "NMT" to represent "no more than" but determined that this particular prescriber used it to communicate "nebulizer mist treatment." Who knows how the patient would have used the hypertonic saline if the pharmacy label had read "Use 4 mL no more than twice daily" rather than "Use 4 mL with nebulizer mist treatment twice daily?"

8. Use of other abbreviations

Some shorthand abbreviations used in prescription can be misinterpreted such as `D/C' for discontinue, death certificate, dilatation and curretage;

`TCA' for to come again, or trichloroacetic acid, or tricyclic antidepressant;

`CST' for continue same treatment, or discontinue 1, 2, 5, rest to continue, symbols '>' and '<', etc. are error prone symbols.

Error proofing examples are shown in box below. Prepare a list of do not use symbols/abbreviations and circulate to all prescribers and staff as applicable.

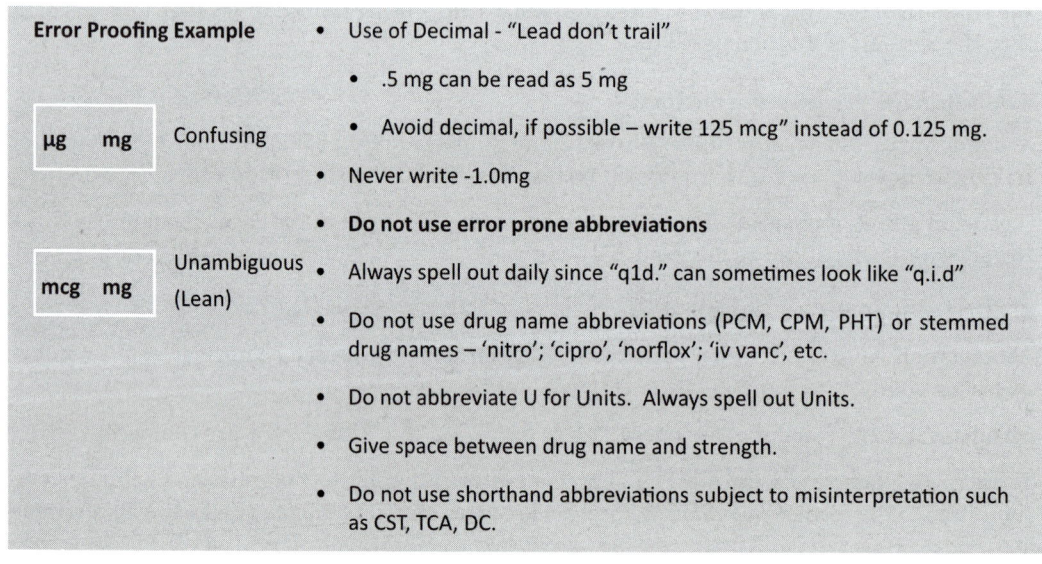

Error Proofing Example		• Use of Decimal - "Lead don't trail"
		• .5 mg can be read as 5 mg
µg mg	Confusing	• Avoid decimal, if possible – write 125 mcg" instead of 0.125 mg.
		• Never write -1.0mg
		• **Do not use error prone abbreviations**
mcg mg	Unambiguous (Lean)	• Always spell out daily since "q1d." can sometimes look like "q.i.d"
		• Do not use drug name abbreviations (PCM, CPM, PHT) or stemmed drug names – 'nitro'; 'cipro', 'norflox'; 'iv vanc', etc.
		• Do not abbreviate U for Units. Always spell out Units.
		• Give space between drug name and strength.
		• Do not use shorthand abbreviations subject to misinterpretation such as CST, TCA, DC.

C. PATIENTS RECEIVING HIGH-ALERT MEDICATIONS

1. High-alert medications are drugs that bear a heightened risk of causing significant patient harm when they are used in error. Although mistakes may or may not be more common with these drugs, the consequences of an error are clearly more devastating to patients. While all drugs, biologics, vaccines, and contrast media have a defined risk profile, concentrated electrolyte solutions for injection are especially dangerous. Reports of death and serious injury/ disability related to the inappropriate administration of these drugs have been continuous and dramatic. Most of the time, it is not clinically possible to reverse the effects of concentrated electrolytes when not administered properly (e.g. not properly diluted, confused with another drug, etc.), and hence, patient death is usually the observed outcome. In short, these agents are deadly when not

prepared and administered properly. Drugs more likely to be involved in serious medication errors are shown below:

> ### Drugs more likely to be involved in serious medication errors
>
> Adrenergic agonists (e.g., epinephrine, phenylephrine, norepinephrine)
>
> IV adrenergic antagonists (e.g., propranolol, metoprolol, labetalol)
>
> Antithrombotic agents & Anticoagulants including warfarin, low-molecular-weight heparin, IV unfractionated heparin, Factor Xa inhibitors (fondaparinux), direct thrombin inhibitors (e.g., argatroban, lepirudin, bivalirudin), thrombolytics (e.g., alteplase, reteplase, tenecteplase), and glycoprotein IIb/IIIa inhibitors (e.g., eptifibatide)
>
> Chemotherapy
>
> Chloral hydrate/midazolam liquid in children
>
> Dextrose, hypertonic, 20% or greater
>
> Concentrated electrolytes
>
> Hypoglycemic agents and Insulin
>
> Inotropic medications, IV (e.g., digoxin, milrinone)
>
> Anesthetic agents, general, inhaled and IV (e.g., propofol, ketamine)
>
> Neuromuscular blocking agents (e.g., succinylcholine, rocuronium, vecuronium)
>
> Opiates IV, transdermal, and oral (including liquid concentrates, immediate and sustained-release formulations)
>
> Theophylline
>
> Radiocontrast agents, IV

2. It is especially critical that the availability, access, prescribing, ordering, preparation, distribution, labeling, verification, administration, and monitoring of these agents be planned in such a way that possible adverse events can be avoided, and, hopefully, be eliminated.

3. This list of high-alert medicines is used to determine which medications require special safeguards to reduce the risk of errors. This may include strategies like:

   i. Improving access to information about these drugs;

   ii. Limiting access to high-alert medications;

   iii. Using auxiliary labels and automated alerts;

   iv. Standardizing the ordering, storage, preparation, and administration of these products;

   v. Controlling availability of these drugs to restricted areas;

   vi. Employing redundancies such as automated or independent double-checks when necessary.

4. Standardizing the dosing, units of measure, and terminology are critical elements of safe use of concentrated electrolyte solutions. Moreover, mix-ups of specific concentrated electrolyte solutions must be avoided (e.g. confusing sodium chloride with potassium chloride). These efforts require special attention, appropriate expertise, inter- professional collaboration, processes of verification, and several forcing functions that would ensure safe use.

D. PATIENTS RECEIVING HIGH-RISK MEDICINES

High risk medications are medicines that present a high risk when administered by the wrong route or when other system errors occur and are involved in a high percentage of medication errors/ sentinel events/high risk for abuse, error or other adverse outcomes, e.g. medications with a low therapeutic index (lithium, digoxin, phenytoin, carbamazepine, valproic acid, phenobarbitone), NDPS/ENDs, psychotherapeutic medications and look-alike, sound-alike (LASA) medicines.

IV. SAFE PRACTICE RECOMMENDATIONS AND ROLE OF PHARMACIST IN PREVENTING ERRORS

Prescribers, pharmacy personnel, and patients have roles in preventing these errors and resultant harm due to errors.

1. Ensure correct entry of the prescription. Pharmacist should be trained to follow good dispensing practices.

2. Confirm that the prescription is correct and complete. Follow all the steps involved in dispensing such as receiving and validating prescription, understanding and interpreting prescription, preparing items for issue, recording action taken and issue medicines to patients with clear instruction and advice. While assessing prescriptions:

    i. Clarify illegible handwriting, nonstandard abbreviations, or incomplete information, if any

    ii. Analyze patient's profile

    iii. Review drug interactions and allergies

    iv. Verify appropriateness of medication and dosage

    v. Consider computer alerts

    vi. Highlight unusual dosage form or strength

3. Beware of Look-alike, Sound-alike (LASA) drugs and eliminate or reduce LASA on your formulary by following:

    i. Identify and, at a minimum, perform annualy review of a list of look-alike/sound-alike drugs including all dosage forms such as tablets, capsules, injection, etc.

    ii. Minimize LASA on your formulary. For example. Heparin 1000 IU/ml and 5000 IU/ml vials are similar looking vials. Select and keep only one dosage form (i.e., either 1000 IU/ml or 5000 IU/ml vial) in inventory to avoid errors.

    iii. Use reminders such as labels and computer notes to prevent mix-ups between "look-alike" and "sound-alike" drug names.

4. **Auxiliary Labelling**[9] Auxiliary labels are generally small stickers consisting of pictogram or one or more letters or lines of text intended to enhance identification, patient knowledge, Identify high-alert/high-risk medicines or medicines which require special precautions using auxiliary labels such as 'Dilute before Use'; 'For External Use Only'; 'Shake Well'; 'Take With Food'; 'Sound-alike'; 'Do NOT Refrigerate'; 'Keep Frozen'; 'Protect from Light', etc (see below).

5. Do not take or minimize verbal/telephone orders for high alert and LASA medicines as drug orders given orally can be misunderstood. Develop policy for verbal orders (see below).

6. Be careful with zeros and abbreviations. Mathematical errors and decimal point misplacement are common causes of errors, especially in conversions between micrograms and milligrams. To prevent confusion and reduce the risk of medication errors, ambiguous abbreviations, including drug name abbreviations, should never be used when communicating drug and patient information.

---

9 An auxiliary label, also called cautionary or advisory label, is a label added on to a dispensed medication package by a pharmacist in addition to the usual prescription label. These labels are intended to provide supplementary information regarding safe administration, use, and storage of the medication.

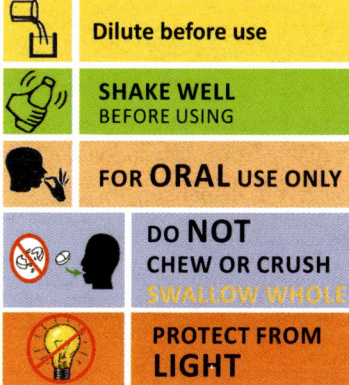

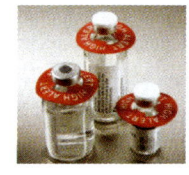
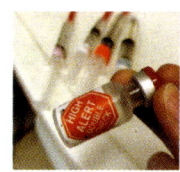
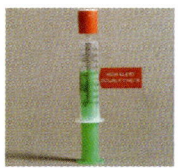
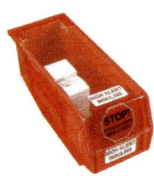
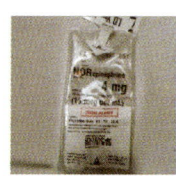

7. Oral liquid medications can be dispensed improperly because of misunderstandings with reading and labeling of oral syringes or use of such devices by parents of pediatric patients. Use appropriate devices for oral liquid medications. See Chapter on dispensing procedures.

8. Pharmacist should check with prescriber before substituting generic as well as branded product.

9. Organize the workplace. Take time to store drugs properly. Practice of cutting strips combined with bad storage increases the chances of dispensing errors.

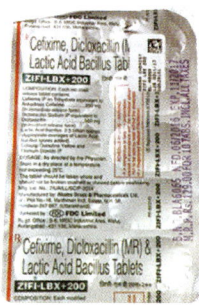
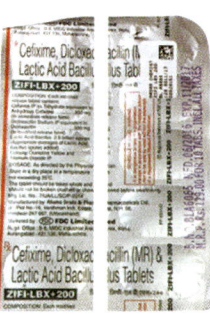
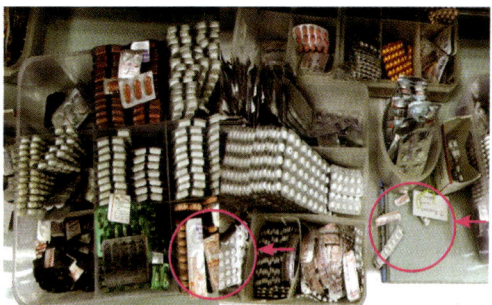

Strip cutting and bad storage – loss of essential information on dose strength, type of dosage form, expiry date, batch no., etc. and also lead to errors due to medicine mix-up especially if there are look alikes of the medicines in stock

10. Thoroughly check all prescriptions. Repeated checking and counter checking. Keep the original prescription order, label, and medication container together throughout the dispensing process. Perform a check on the contents of prescription and containers. Compare the contents of the medication container with the information on the prescription label. Perform a final check on the prescription label. When possible, use automation, such as bar coding.

11. Always provide thorough patient counselling.
    i. Make sure drug references in the pharmacy are current;
    ii. At minimum, double check all calculations;
    iii. Have all prescriptions double checked by another person, if possible

12. Reduce distraction when possible. Focus on reducing stress and balancing heavy workloads.

13. Be careful with Computerised Physician Order Entry (CPOE): Though CPOE improves communication and reduces some types of errors but, this technology may have its own pitfalls:
    i. Lower case L may look like the numeral 1

  ii. Letter O may look like the numeral 0 (zero)

  iii. Letter Z and the numeral 2 may be misread

  iv. Wrong patient or wrong drug chosen from list

14. Use Computerised alerts . Computer systems can be configured to flash maximum dose alerts and other safety alerts. Upgrades are necessary and usually available from software vendors.

  Optimal capabilities of pharmacy computer software alerts to prevent dispensing include:

  i. Dose limits   ii. Allergic reactions   iii. Cross-allergies

  iv. Duplication of drug ingredients   v. Drug interactions

  vi. Contraindicated drugs or drugs that need dosage modifications

V. POLICY FOR VERBAL/TELEPHONE ORDERS

1. Avoid when possible – preferably orders to be taken by Resident Doctors/ Medical Officer (MOs). In emergency situations or some special situations only the following personnel may be authorized to accept verbal/telephone orders:

   Registered Nurse, Certified Nurse Practitioner, Clinical Nurse Specialist, Registered Pharmacist

2. The above personnel may take and implement the verbal/telephone order within the scope of their practice, education, and licensure. The individual accepting the verbal/telephone order is responsible for alerting the medical staff to co-sign the order. The person accepting the verbal/phone order should flag the unsigned paper order in the medical record.

3. Verbal/telephone orders should not be accepted for some categories of orders such as:

   i. Chemotherapy treatment (except holding of treatment)

   ii. Patient controlled analgesia (PCAs) (except minor changes or clarifications)

   iii. Withdrawal of life support

   iv. Hyperalimentation [10] (except minor changes or clarifications)

   v. Intraspinal opioid orders

4. Verbal/telephone orders for patient restraints must comply with hospital policy.

5. When calling in a telephone order, confirm patient identity, particularly when the telephone call is unexpected or not initiated by the practitioners in the unit or caring for the patient. Use at least two patient identifiers. If possible identify by any unique feature. Do not use bed number or room number for identification.

6. Verbal/telephone orders relating to medications should include the name of the patient, date and time of the order, drug name, dosage, route, frequency, name of the ordering physician and, if applicable, indication for PRN use and duration.

7. Ensure all telephone orders are complete (i.e., include the "five rights": patient name, medication, dose, time(s)/frequency, and route).

8. Record the order directly onto an order sheet in the patient's chart as the order is received. (Be prepared when calling a physician for the possibility of a telephone order to be received. Do not write orders on a scrap piece of paper as transferring this information introduces another opportunity for error).

9. Enunciate slowly and distinctly.

10. Read back all telephone orders or test results. Some hospital policies require the practitioner to indicate, as part of the written telephone order that a *read back* has occurred.

---

10 Hyperalimentation is artificial supply of nutrients by IV route such as total parenteral nutrition.

11. Read back should include:

    i. Spelling of drug name (vi. High alert drugs use words to identify letters that are phonetically similar e.g., "B as in Bombay" versus "V as in Varanasi"), may include trade name if this helps with clarity especially when telephone orders involve LASA and high alert medication.

    ii. State numbers like pilots as an order for "NPH insulin 16 units" can easily sound like "NPH insulin 60 units." One-five mg for 15 mg; Dose confirmation expressed as a single digit (e.g., "fifty milligrams: five, zero, milligrams")

    iii. If a dosage range is ordered, Order for Digoxin 0.125 mg, may be heard and transcribed as a dose range of ".1 - 5 mg", telephone order for 'fentanyl drip transcribed as 5,200 mcg per hour, however, intended order was for a fentanyl drip 50 to 100 mcg per hour, therefore, include this in the verification e.g., "dosage range of fifty micrograms: five, zero, micrograms per hour up to and including one hundred: one, zero, zero, micrograms per hour intravenously".

    iv. Specify concentration instead of giving the dose in number of teaspoonful, tablets, ampoules or vials especially preparation which come in several dosage forms such as Paracetamol / Iron preparations.

12. Avoid truncating, using abbreviations, short forms or acronyms for drug names to avoid confusion e.g., state "morphine" rather than "morph", "hydrocholorothiazide rather than "HCTZ", it can be mistaken for hydrocortisone; "potassium chloride" rather than "K", it can be mistaken for Vitamin K.

13. Avoid abbreviations for the dose frequency e.g., state "three times a day" instead of "tid", or "every eight hours" instead of "q8h".

14. Provide complete dosage and route for all medications ordered and comply with formulary guidelines e.g., mmol for potassium; mg; mcg; mcg/kg/min; mg/kg/hour; mg rather than ml for oral suspensions; include infusion volume when applicable.

15. Verify indication for medication(s) ordered. The order needs to make sense according to the treatment plan for the patient. Ask questions as needed e.g., clarification, any concerns.

16. Consider review by a second practitioner before initiating an order, particularly for medications available in unit stock or when an over-ride is required to access a medication especially from an automated dispensing unit.

17. When pharmacy is expected to fill an order, a copy of the written order should be sent for review *before* the medication is dispensed. Copies of all orders should be sent to pharmacy to ensure a complete and upto-date pharmacy medication record. This provides the opportunity for another check to prevent or limit perpetuation of an error, drug interactions, allergies, duplicate therapies, etc.

18. Call the practitioner back if any questions or discrepancies arise e.g., incomplete order noted, unusual dosage, etc.

19. After confirming accuracy of order, recipient of order should sign order as transcriber stating 'as per Dr....... Instructions'. Verbal/telephone orders must include the date, time and name of the ordering practitioner and the name of the person writing or entering the order.

20. Verbal/telephone orders must be authenticated by the practitioner within twelve (12) hours of issuing order. If a physician is off duty or away and thus cannot sign within the aforementioned time limit, a covering physician may sign the verbal/telephone order and assumes responsibility for his/her colleague's order as being complete.

4 | Adverse Drug Reaction Reporting

Adverse drug reactions (ADRs) are the leading cause of morbidity, mortality and increased healthcare cost. Despite drastic improvement in healthcare practices, ADRs are contributing towards poor clinical outcome, hospitalization, prolongation of hospital stay, and enhanced economic burden. All drugs are capable of producing adverse effects. Adverse effects may develop immediately or only after prolonged use of drug. ADRs are more common with multiple drug therapy and in elderly patients. Chances of some ADR increase when drug is given for a long time or if patient is suffering from allergic diseases. There is very limited information available in India on ADR. It has been estimated that 30–50% ADRs are preventable. An incidence of 10–25% has been documented in different clinical settings.

I. DEFINITIONS

Adverse event: It is defined as any untoward medical occurrence that may be present during treatment with a medicine but which does not necessarily have a causal relationship with this treatment.

Adverse drug reactions (ADRs): It is a response to a medicine which is noxious and unintended and which occurs at doses normally used in man (WHO). It does not include therapeutic failures, overdose, drug abuse, non-compliance and medication errors.

Side effect: It is any unintended effect other than the intended therapeutic effect, whether beneficial, neutral or harmful) with a pharmaceutical product occurring at doses normally used by a patient that is related to the pharmacological properties of the drug. Side effects and ADRs often are used interchangeably.

A serious adverse event or serious adverse drug reaction is "any untoward medical occurrence that at any dose:

1. Result in death
2. Is life threatening
3. Requires hospitalization or prolongation of existing hospitalization
4. Results in persistent or significant disability/incapacity
5. Is a congenital anomaly/birth defect".

II. CLASSIFICATION OF ADRs

Adverse drug reactions can be categorized in a number of ways (e.g. duration incidence/frequency, by severity, types of ADRs, location and by body systems affected). The following categorization is often used:

A. BASED ON TYPES OF ADRs

ADRs have been broadly classified into:

1. **Type A (Augmented) Reactions:** Are those related to the exaggerated pharmacological

effects of the drugs and tend to be fairly common (usually more than 1 in 100), often predictable and dose dependent (more frequent and more severe at higher dosage) and may often be avoided by using dosages that are appropriate for the individual patients, e.g. hypoglycaemia with insulin, hypotension with antihypertensive agent, constipation with morphine, bleeding with anticoagulants, bradycardia with beta blockers, headache with nitrates, postural hypotension with prazosin, etc. Type A reactions are usually reproducible and can be studied experimentally and have high morbidity but low mortality.

2. **Type B (Bizarre) reactions:** Are those that are unexpected and unpredictable and often related to patient factors like genetic predisposition, allergy, etc. They occur in a minority of the patients (less than 1 per 100), are often serious, may show little or no relationship with dosage and may be difficult to predict. These reactions can be precipitated by small amounts of drugs and repeated exposure will cause recurrence of reactions. Often include skin rash, angioneurotic oedema, serum sickness and anaphylaxis or asthma. These reactions are often suspected with their relationship to time but have a low background frequency.

Hypersensitivity: A term sometime used interchangeably with drug allergy is the result of antigen—antibody reactions that occur in the body. One of the most dangerous of all drug hypersensitive reactions is penicillin allergy. In its more severe form, penicillin anaphylaxis becomes fatal. One should always remain well prepared to face anaphylaxis as anaphylaxis on one hand is fatal, but patient can be saved if right drug is administered immediately, i.e. Adrenaline. Parental administration of drugs carries greater risk of acute hypersensitivity reactions than oral administration.

 i. *Common cutaneous allergic reactions include:* Exanthema, urticaria, contact dermatitis, and fixed drug eruptions

 ii. More serious and potentially fatal forms of drug rashes/hypersensitivity reactions include Toxic Epidermal Necrolysis (TEN), Stevens-Johnson syndrome and drug hypersensitivity syndrome. These are potentially life-threatening with significant morbidity, if not recognized and treated in time. Drug hypersensitivity syndrome is characterised by fever, rash and internal organ involvement. Prompt diagnosis is vital, along with identification and early withdrawal of suspect medicines. Avoidance of re-exposure to the responsible agent is essential. Cross-reactivity to structurally related medicines is common. First-degree relatives may be predisposed to developing this syndrome.

 iii. *Rarely*: Idiosyncratic reaction occurs. These are highly unpredictable, individual and unusual. One of the best-known idiosyncratic reaction is chloramphenicol induced aplastic anaemia which occurs 1 in 40,000 patients. Although rare but when occurs, it is mostly fatal.

3. *Type C (Chronic) reactions:* These are associated with long-term use of a drug and involves dose accumulation, e.g. ototoxicity, renal toxicity caused by aminoglycoside, analgesic nephropathy interstitial nephritis caused by phenacetin, ocular toxicity caused by antimalarials, visual disturbances with ethambutol, tardive dyskinesia with neuroleptics, etc.

4. *Type D (Delayed) reactions:* These are delayed effects (dose independent), timing makes it more difficult to detect, e.g.—leucopenia after weeks of use of lomustine, teratogenesis, e.g. foetal hydantoin syndrome with phenytoin, carcinogenesis like clear cell carcinoma of the female reproductive tract in matured women whose mothers have received diethylstilbestrol during pregnancy.

5. *Type E (End of use) reactions:* Which occur when the discontinuation of the drug is too abrupt, especially after long term therapy with the drug e.g. adrenocortical insufficiency due to sudden withdrawal of corticosteroids, rebound hypertension after sudden withdrawal of Clonidine.

B. BASED ON DURATION

Temporary, persistent or permanent.

C. BASED ON INCIDENCE (FREQUENCY OF OCCURRENCE)

1. Very common (>1/10 patients)
2. Common (>1/100)
3. Uncommon (>1/1000)
4. Rare (>1/10,000)
5. Very rare (1/100,000).

III. SEVERITY ASSESSMENT OF ADRs

Mild: ADR considered mild when it does not interfere with daily routine of the patient or need any treatment, viz., slight sedation with antihistamines.

Moderate: ADR considered moderate when there is a need to reduce the dose or change the drug or hospital stay is prolonged.

Severe: Severe or medically significant but not immediately life threatening, hospitalization or prolongation of hospitalization indicated, disabling, limiting self care and activities of daily living (ADL). Hypersensitivity reactions leading to anaphylaxis is one of the most severe adverse drug reactions.

Lethal: Life- threatening consequences, urgent intervention is indicated. ADR is considered lethal if it results in death of the patient, i.e., Complete A-V block by digoxin.

IV. CASUALITY ASSESSMENT OF ADRs

The causality (the relationship between cause and effect) assessment is usually based on:

1. The temporal relationship[11] between drug use and the adverse event (challenge, dechallenge and rechallenge).

    i. **Dechallenge:** "Dechallenge" is defined as assessing the resolution of ADR on withdrawal of a drug. If ADR disappears after withdrawal of drug dechallenge is considered as positive.

    ii. **Rechallenge:** "Rechallenge" is defined as assessing the appearance of ADR on reinstitution of drug. If ADR appears after reinstitution of drug, rechallenge is considered to be positive. Rechallenge routinely not performed; if required it should only be performed under supervision of the doctor.

2. The established knowledge about the drug, i.e., its actions, kinetics, and adverse effects.

3. Characteristic clinical and laboratory findings.

4. Likelihood of exclusion of other explanations.

5. The data, so analyzed, is put into various causal categories to describe whether the implicated drug is indeed responsible for the reaction or not. These categories, as described by the WHO are:

    i. **Certain:** A clinical event, including laboratory test abnormality occurring in a plausible time relationship to drug administration, and which cannot be explained by concurrent disease or other drugs or chemicals. The response to withdrawal of the drug (dechallenge) and reintroduction of the drug (rechallenge) should be positive.

    ii. **Probable/Likely:** A clinical event, including laboratory test abnormality, with a reasonable time sequence to administration of the drug, unlikely to be attributed to

---

11 A temporal relationship is the timing between a factor and an outcome which can be used to assign causality to a relationship.

concurrent disease or other drugs or chemicals, and which follows a clinically reasonable response to withdrawal (dechallenge) is positive. Rechallenge information is not necessary in this category.

iii. **Possible:** A clinical event, including laboratory test abnormality, with a reasonable time sequence to administration of the drug, but which could also be explained by concurrent disease or other drugs or chemicals, information on de-challenge is lacking or unclear.

V. FACTORS CONTRIBUTING TO ADRs

Factors contributing to the adverse reactions are numerous and most are avoidable. It is necessary to take, or try to take into account, which effects are avoidable (by skilled choice and use) and which are unavoidable (inherent in drug or the patient) so that rational and safe use of drugs can be made.

1. An error in diagnosing the disease.
2. Prescription of the wrong drug for the right disease.
3. Prescription of the wrong dose of right drug.
4. The drug is right for the disease but wrong for the patient due to a genetic or ethnic predisposition, age, some other illness (like renal failure) or medication, allergy or intolerance.
5. Noncompliance on part of patient.
6. Self medication by the patient.
7. Taking of many drugs (polypharmacy) or receiving treatment from more than one source (polytherapy).
8. Counterfeit drugs
9. Poor quality of pharmaceutical products.

ADRs occurring due to medication errors, drug-drug/drug-food interaction are usually preventable. These can be prevented, if the physician/pharmacist is having adequate knowledge about the drug interactions and adverse effects of the prescribed drugs.

Relationship between Adverse events, adverse drug reactions and near miss

Chart indicates penicillin allergy but penicillin ordered, given and patient has severe reaction

Adverse Drug Reaction | Adverse event | No Harm/near Miss

No history of penicillin allergy; penicillin ordered, given & patient has allergic reaction | Penicillin given at a dose of 500mg when 250mg ordered and patient progresses as expected

VI. PREVENTION AND DEALING WITH ADRs

Though ADRs cannot be prevented to a level of 100%. However, several studies have shown that 35-50% ADRs can be prevented. Hence, preventing ADR is another step for ensuring medication safety in patients.

1. Avoid inappropriate use of drugs, consider possible duplication or drug-drug interactions when new drug added to prescription.
2. Use appropriate dose, route, frequency based on patient's need.
3. Elicit history of allergy to drugs and allergic diseases viz., asthma, food allergy.
4. Adopt correct drug administration technique, e.g., NSAID to be given after meals.
5. Appropriate laboratory test monitoring as may be required.
6. To deal with ADR correctly, one needs to be alert to even minor changes in patient's clinical status.
   i. Listen to patient's minor complaint. Such minor complaints may be warning for future reactions.
   ii. One may reduce dose after consulting prescriber or reschedule dose.

iii. Inform patients what ADRs to expect, so that patient does not get worried, otherwise may stop taking drug. e.g., black stools with iron, orange discolouration of body fluids, urine with rifampicin.

Some ADRs are dose related and disappear as dose is reduced and some subside with continuous use, e.g., drowsiness with paroxetine, cough with enalapril. Patient may develop tolerance to some ADRs such as headache with amlodepine. However, few ADRs are hazardous and unacceptable, require discontinuation of drug.

iv. Always advise patient to report ADR to prescriber, pharmacist or nurse immediately.

v. If severe reaction is suspected, withhold drug and check with prescriber.

VII. REPORTING OF ADRs

1. Reporting of ADRs can prevent developing tragedies with new medicines. Medicines have been withdrawn from the market on the basis of ADR reporting, viz. Thalidomide induced phocomelia; Terfenadine induced fatal cardiac arrhythmias; Temafloxacin induced hemolytic anaemia; Rofecoxib induced cardiac arrhythmias.

2. *Post-marketing surveillance is important to permit detection of less common, but sometimes very serious ADRs. Therefore, health professionals should report ADRs as it can save lives of their patients and others.*

3. All health care workers, including doctors, dentists, pharmacists, nurses and other health professionals should report all suspected adverse reactions to drugs (including vaccines, X-ray contrast media, traditional and herbal remedies), especially when the reaction is unusual, potentially serious or clinically significant. It is vital to report an adverse drug reaction to the Drug Regulatory Authority, Pharmacoviglance programme even if one does not have all the facts or are uncertain that the medicine is definitely responsible for causing the reaction.

4. Adverse drug reaction must be reported to the patient's medical practitioner, as well as to Drugs Control Authority.

5. Adverse drug reactions to the Drug Regulatory Authority's Pharmacoviglance Programme (PvPI) using (Suspected ADR reporting form available on http://www.cdsco.nic.in/writereaddata/ADR%20form%20PvPI.pdf) or dial toll free helpline number - 1800 180 3024 to report ADRs. Mail filled ADR reporting form directly to pvpi@ipcindia.net or pvpi.ipcindia@gmail.com"

6. ADRs such as below should be reported:

   i. All ADRs to newly marketed drugs or new drugs added to the Essential Drugs List/Hospital Formulary.

   ii. All serious reactions and interactions

   iii. ADRs which are not clearly stated in the package insert

   iv. Unusual or interesting adverse drug reactions

   v. All adverse reactions or poisonings to traditional or herbal remedies

7. In addition to above, report product quality problems such as:

   i. Suspected contamination

   ii. Questionable stability

   iii. Defective components

   iv. Poor packaging or labelling

   v. Therapeutic failures.

SUSPECTED ADVERSE DRUG REACTION REPORTING FORM

For VOLUNTARY reporting of Adverse Drug Reactions by healthcare professionals

CDSCO **Central Drugs Standard Control Organization** Directorate General of Health Services, Ministry of Health & Family Welfare, Government of India, FDA Bhavan, ITO, Kotla Road, New Delhi www.cdsco.nic.in	**(AMC/ NCC Use only)** AMC Report No. Worldwide Unique no.

A. Patient Information

1.Patient Initials _____	2.Age at time of Event or date of birth --------------------	3. Sex ☐M ☐ F 4. Weight _____Kgs

B .Suspected Adverse Reaction

5. Date of reaction stated (dd/mm/yyyy)

6. Date of recovery (dd/mm/yyyy)

7. Describe reaction or problem

12. Relevant tests / laboratory data with dates

13. Other relevant history including pre-existing medical conditions (e.g. allergies, race, pregnancy, smoking, alcohol use, hepatic/ renal dysfunction etc)

14. Seriousness of the reaction

☐ Death (dd/mm/yyy)____   ☐ Congenitial anomaly
☐ Life threatening   ☐ Required intervention
☐ Hospitalization-initial or   to prevent permanent
   prolonged   impairment / damage
☐ Disability   ☐ Other (specify)

15. Outcomes

☐ Fatal   ☐ Recovering   ☐ Unknown
☐ Continuing   ☐ Recovered   ☐Other (specify)____

C.Suspected medication(s)

S.No	8. Name (brand and /or generic name)	Manufacturer (if known)	Batch No./ Lot No. (if known)	Exp. Date (if known)	Dose used	Route used	Frequency	Therapy dates (if known give duration)		Reason for use of prescribed for
								Date started	Date stopped	
i.										
ii.										
iii.										
iv.										

Sl.No As per C	9. Reaction abated after drug stopped or dose reduced					10. Reaction reappeared after reintroduction				
	Yes	No	Unknown	NA	Reduced dose	Yes	No	Unknown	NA	If reintroduced dose
i.										
ii.										
iii.										
iv.										

11. Concomitant medical product including self medication and herbal remedies with therapy dates (exclude those used to treat reaction)

D. Reporter (see confidentiality section in first page)

16. Name and Professional Address :_____
_____
Pin code : _____ E-mail _____
Tel. No. (with STD code): _____
Occupation _____Signature _____

17. Causality Assessment	18. Date of this report (dd/mm/yyyy)

ADVICE ABOUT REPORTING

- Report adverse experiences with medications
- Report serious adverse reactions. A reaction is serious when the patient outcome is:

  - death
  - life-threatening (real risk of dying)
  - hospitalization (initial or prolonged)
  - disability (significant, persistent or permanent
  - congenital anomaly
  - required intervention to prevent permanent impairment or damage

- **Report even if:**

  - You're not certain the product caused adverse reaction
  - you don't have all the details, however, point nos. **1, 5, 7, 8, 11, 15, 16 & 18** (see reverse) are essentially required.

- **Who can report:**

  - Any health care professional (Doctors including Dentists, Nurses and Pharmacists)

- **Where to report:**

  - Please return the completed form to the nearest *Adverse drug reaction Monitoring Centre (AMC)* or to *National Coordinating Centre*
  - A list of nationwide AMCs is available at: http://cdsco.nic.in/pharmacovigilance.htm

- **What happens to the submitted information:**

  - Information provided in this form is handled in strict confidence. The causality assessment is carried out at Adverse Drug Reaction Monitoring Centres (AMCs) by using WHO-UMC scale. The analyzed forms are forwarded to the National Coordinating Centre through the ADR database. Finally the data is analyzed and forwarded to the Global Pharmacovigilance Database managed by WHO Uppsala Monitoring Center in Sweden.

  - The reports are periodically reviewed by the National Coordinating Centre (PvPI) The information generated on the basis of these reports helps in continuous assessment of the benefit-risk ratio of medicines.

  - The information is submitted to the Steering Committee of PvPI constituted by the Ministry of Health and Family Welfare. The Committee is entrusted with the responsibility to review the data and suggest any interventions that may be required.

Suspected Adverse Drug Reaction Reporting Form

For VOLUNTARY reporting of suspected adverse drug reactions by health care professionals

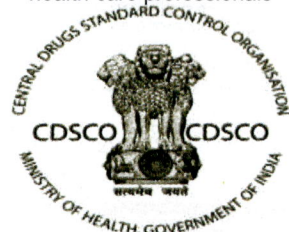

Central Drugs Standard Control Organization
Directorate General of Health Services,
Ministry of Health & Family Welfare, Government of India
FDA Bhawan, ITO Kotla Road, New Delhi – 110002
www.cdsco.nic.in

Pharmacovigilance
Programme
of
India
for
Assuring Drug
Safety

Pharmacovigilance Programme of India (PvPI)

National Coordinating Centre,
Indian Pharmacopoeia Commission
Ministry of Health & Family Welfare,
Govt. of India
Sector 23, Raj Nagar, Ghaziabad-201 002.Tel.:0120-2783400, 2783401, 2783392, FAX: 0120-2783311
E.mail: ipclab@vsnl.net

Confidentiality: The patient's identity is held in strict confidence and protected to the fullest extent. Programme staff is not ex- pected to and will not disclose the reporter's identity in response to a request from the public. **Submission of a report does not constitute an admission that medical personnel or manufacturer or the product caused or contributed to the reaction.**

5 | Pharmaceutical Supply Management

The supply and management of drugs is a continuous process that involves selection of medicines, their actual needs, procurement, storage/distribution and use. Each of the steps in the management cycle needs to be monitored with the aim of improving all its elements addressing following issues:

1. Selection of well documented quality products from reliable manufacturers.

2. Certificate of analysis of delivered products

3. Use of Good Manufacturing Practices certificate

4. Quality assessment of drugs upon receipt

5. Inspection of shipments

6. Independent laboratory testing for quality assurance

7. Appropriate storage and transport

8. Appropriate dispensing and use

9. Monitoring of product quality/reporting system.

The pharmaceutical staff performs a variety of tasks to handle following duties which may vary according to the capacity, staff, size, etc:

- Selection of drugs

- Management of the Essential medicines

- Estimation of medicine needs

- Procurement

- Distribution and storage

- Rational use of medicines

The following chapters describe each of these functions in detail.

I. HOSPITAL FORMULARY

Credibility, effectiveness and attendance at health services, depend on a large extent on patient being able to obtain relevant drugs at the right time. No hospital pharmacy can possibly stock every medication that its affiliated doctors may want to prescribe for their hospitalized patients. Consequently, the medical and pharmacy staffs of hospitals compose a hospital formulary, which is a list of the medications that the hospital pharmacy stocks, along with information about each medication.

Formulary system is a mechanism for ongoing assessment of medications that are available for use to assure the safe and effective use of drugs in a cost conscious manner and is the cornerstone of good pharmaceutical management & safe use of medicines.

A formulary list (Also referred as Essential Medicines List [EML]) consists of the most cost-effective, safe, locally available drugs of assured quality that will satisfy the health care needs of the majority of the patients.

A formulary list and formulary manual should be developed and maintained based on recommended treatments from Standard Treatment Guidelines (STGs), using explicit drug selection criteria (relative efficacy, safety, suitability and cost), that have been agreed previously by all departments.

The creation and continuous evaluation of a hospital's formulary facilitates superior patient care, achieves therapeutic goals, and improves patient safety while curtailing expenses.

The Pharmacy and Therapeutics Committee (PTC) or Drugs & Therapeutic Committee (DTC) of a hospital is responsible for compiling, maintaining and updating its formulary. The committee consists of a representative clinician from major specialties, a nurse, a store in-charge/pharmacist, an administrator (representing the hospital administration or finance department), clinical microbiologist, a clinical pharmacologist, if available and a member of the hospital records department. A dedicated and committed chairperson and secretary are critical to the success and efficiency of a DTC. The committee chooses medications based on their effectiveness, their cost and the need for them at each particular hospital. For instance, a small community hospital would not include an expensive cancer chemotherapy drug in its formulary, whereas a major cancer center would include several such medications.

II. DEFINITIONS

Essential Medicines: These medicines are those that satisfy priority need of majority of patients in a hospital and should be available to patients at all times. These are selected with due regards to disease prevalence in a hospital.

Essential medicines concept is based on the principle that a limited number of drugs lead to

1. A better supply of drugs
2. More rational prescribing
3. Procurement of good quality drugs at lower costs
4. Easier storage, distribution and dispensing
5. Focused training and drug information
6. Prescribers gain more experience with fewer drugs and recognize ADR better.

Drug formulary: A formulary is a continually updated list of medications and related information available for use at a hospital or health-system, representing the clinical judgment of physicians, pharmacists, and other experts in the diagnosis and/or treatment of disease and promotion of health. This list includes the dosage forms, strengths and package sizes of each of the medications on it.

Closed formulary: A list of medications (formulary) limiting access of a prescriber to the medicines on this list only. e.g., antibiotics for ICU only, medicines to be prescribed by specialist only.

Non-formulary agent: A medication that is not a part of the drug formulary. This may be due to the medication not being considered for formulary addition or the medication being considered but the DTC choosing not to add it. However, exclusion from the Essential Medicines List/formulary does not imply that no other drugs are useful, but inclusion simply means that in a given situation these drugs are needed for the health care of the majority of the population.

Therapeutic class review: An evaluation of a group of medications with an established therapeutic class (e.g., first-generation cephalosporins; NSAIDs- Non-Steroidal Anti Inflammatory Drugs; anti-hypertensives). The review evaluates the indications for use, pharmacokinetics/dynamics, adverse effects, drug interactions, dosage regimens, and cost to determine similarities and differences between the therapeutic classes.

Therapeutic equivalent: Drug products with different chemical structures but of the same pharmacologic or therapeutic class and usually having similar therapeutic effects and adverse-reaction profiles when administered to patients in therapeutically equivalent doses. e.g., first generation cephalosporins; histamine-2 blockers such as ranitidine, famotidine, nizatidine; Angiotensin Converting Enzyme Inhibitors (ACEIs) –enalapril, ramipril, lisinopril and Angiotensin Receptor Blocker (ARB) - losartan, telmisartan, valsarten; HMG-CoA Reductase Inhibitors or "Statins" rosuvastatin, atorvastatin, simvastatin, lovastatin, pravastatin, etc.

Therapeutic interchange or the generic substitution: These are the authorized exchange of therapeutic alternatives in accordance with previously established and approved written guidelines or protocols within formulary system. Establishment of therapeutic equivalents extends beyond the chemical entity. It must include the dosage strength, dose frequency, and route of administration for the interchange. E.g., diclofenac 50 mg three times a day may be therapeutically interchanged with diclofenac SR 75 mg.

Formulary restrictions: The act of limiting the use of specific formulary medications to specific physicians based on:

   i   Areas of expertise (e.g., cardiology),

   ii   Patient disease state (e.g., acute myocardial infarction), or

   iii   Location (e.g., operating room, ICU, etc.).

   iv   High-end antibiotics to ICUs, concentrated electrolytes restricted to OTs and ICUs, chemotherapeutic medicines to oncology wards only and similarly restrictions on, high-risk medicines.

III. DEVELOPING HOSPITAL FORMULARY

1. It is a primary responsibility of hospital Drugs & Therapeutics Committee (DTC).

2. DTC should develop hospitals' own formulary giving due consideration to national / state EML and consideration to national / hospital treatment protocols viz. malaria, TB, etc.

3. Establish a transparent process for creating and updating the list of essential medicines, provide a voice for key stakeholders, but ensure a scientific, evidence-based process.

Step 1: Prioritize a list of common problems/diseases being treated in the hospital and determine the first choice of treatment for each problem.

1. The disease may be ranked to identify the most common disease being treated in the hospital by consulting all medical departments and reviewing the previous hospital mortality and morbidity records.

2. For each disease, identify an appropriate first choice of treatment using Standard Treatment Guidelines (STGs) either nationally or locally developed. Alternatively, an expert committee can be brought together to identify the appropriate treatment for each of the common health problems.

3. Select medicines as per criteria given below:

   i. *Choice of drugs depending on: the* pattern of prevalent diseases, available treatment facilities, training experience of the available personnel, financial resources, genetic, demographic and environmental factors

   ii. Criteria for selection of Essential Medicines:

   a. Select essential medicines on the basis of efficacy, safety, suitability and cost. Select only those drugs for which sound and adequate data on efficacy, safety are available and for which evidence of performance in general use in a variety of medical settings has been obtained.

   b. Each selected medicine must be available in a form in which adequate quality, including bioavailability, can be assured; its stability under the anticipated conditions of storage and use must be established.

   c. When two or more medicines appear to be similar in the above respects, the choice between them should be made on the basis of a careful evaluation of their relative efficacy, safety, quality, price and availability.

   d. In cost comparison between medicines, the cost of the total treatment, and not only the unit cost of the medicine, must be considered. Where drugs are not entirely similar, selection should be made on the basis of a cost-effectiveness analysis.

   e. In some cases, the choice may also be influenced by other factors, such as pharmacokinetic properties, or by local considerations such as the availability of facilities for storage or manufacturer.

   f. Most essential medicines should be formulated as single compounds. Fixed-ratio combination products are acceptable only when the dosage of each ingredient meets the requirements of a defined population and when the combination has a proven advantage over single compounds administered separately in therapeutic effect, safety or compliance.

   g. Drugs are specified by the international nonproprietary name (INN) or generic name without reference to brand names as far as possible or specific manufacturers depending on the hospital policy.

Step 2: Draft, circulate for comment, and finalize the formulary list

1. Prepare a draft of the list with formulary listing including the therapeutic category– such as anti-neoplastic agent for cancer drugs – of each drug that it carries, followed by its generic and trade names. The listing also includes its dosage form, strength, packing unit, and information about how to store, mix and dilute it, if applicable.

2. Prepare a draft of the list and identify:

    i.   The most important medicines (which are absolutely essential) and those that are less essential.

    ii. The most expensive or fast moving medicines

    iii. Whether all the medicines that are prescribed in large volumes, or are expensive, are essential (Develop matrix of ABC analysis and VED analysis- for details see chapter on quantification of medicine needs and inventory management).

3. Each department, whether clinical or involved in non-clinical drug management, must be given the chance to comment on the list.

4. DTC must deliberate on their comments and provide feedback.

5. Make all information to be discussed and deliberated upon, such as disease profile and STGs, available during the discussions, together with evidence-based reviews where possible.

6. Discuss and finalize the formulary list.

7. Disseminate the formulary list and the reasons for its choices.

Step 3: Develop policies and guidelines for implementation of a hospital formulary

The formulary list will never be useful unless there are documented policies and guidelines on how it should be used. These should include:

1. Distribute hospital formulary to all its intended users – hard copies/online.

2. Separate lists for different levels of health care (PHCs, CHCs, district hospitals and tertiary care) based on local morbidity patterns to be drawn from the main list at the State level or different patient care areas from the hospital formulary.

3. Determine who all should use the list (prescribers and the procurement department should both abide by the list). Restrict procurement to medicines in the hospital formulary.

4. How the list should be reviewed & updated. A clear mechanism for adding and deleting medicines from the list should be enumerated.

5. Mechanism for sending requests for medicines that are not included on the list in exceptional or emergency situations (for example, certain non-formulary drugs may be prescribed by authorized senior doctors for specified less common conditions on named patient basis).

6. The DTC should establish guidelines for generic substitution and therapeutic interchange, if any required.

7. The pharmacist is responsible for selecting generically equivalent products in concert with Drugs Control Authority Regulations. Prescribers may specify a specific brand, if clinically justified. The decision should be based on pharmacologic and/or therapeutic considerations relative to the patient.

8. The DTC determines therapeutic equivalents and how they are processed.

9. The pharmacist is responsible for the quality, quantity, and source of all medications, chemical, biologicals, and pharmaceutical preparations used in the diagnosis and treatment of patients. Such products should meet the relevant standards of the Indian Pharmacopoeia (IP), United States Pharmacopeia (USP), British Pharmacopoeia (BP).

Step 4: Educate staff about the formulary list and monitor implementation

1. Educate all staff in the hospital including doctors, pharmacists and nurses about the list.

2. Make the list of essential medicines, formulary manuals and clinical guidelines widely available in all health care facilities and to all health care providers in both printed and electronic form.

3. Link the essential medicines list to clinical guidelines for diagnosis and treatment, involving both specialists and primary care providers.

4. Only procure medicines on the hospital formulary. Drugs included in the list should be available in hospital pharmacy all the time.

5. Executive/Administrative orders with instructions to doctors that they are required to prescribe only those drugs on the list.

6. Consider establishing an administrative or budgetary safety valve for the limited supply and use of non-listed medicines, e.g. by certain specialist units. For example the hospitals to be instructed to spend 90% of their drug budget on essential medicines only. However, to allow flexibility, tertiary care and super-specialty hospitals to be provided with a discretionary budget of 10% to procure drugs outside the formulary for special situations.

7. Actively engage support from medical opinion leaders, senior clinicians, training institutions, professional organizations, non-governmental organizations and the public.

8. Make clear the specific legal or administrative authority of the essential medicines list for training, procurement, reimbursement and public information.

9. Consider launching new or revised lists with the involvement of prescribers and other officials. In case of state EML involving government officials, such as the Minister of Health, and intensive press coverage and government order for strict implementation with provision of dealing with violations.

IV. FORMULARY SYSTEM MAINTENANCE: ADDING AND DELETING DRUGS

Formulary maintenance is the ongoing process of assuring relative safety and efficacy of agents available for use in the health-system.

1. Review of the formulary should occur initially frequently (1-2 times per year) but the entire formulary should be reviewed every 2 years whereas clinical guidelines should be reviewed and revised every second year and impact should be monitored.

2. For an efficient formulary management do not passively wait for applications to add new medicines to the formulary.

3. Processes used in formulary maintenance include the following:
   i.   New product evaluation
   ii. Therapeutic class review
   iii. Formulary changes (rationale for retaining or deleting an agent from the formulary)
   iv. Non-formulary drug use review

A. MEDICATION REVIEW PROCESS

1. All applications for addition of medicines to the formulary list must be made on an official application form. Individual doctors making an application must get the endorsement of their head of department. Standard format for new drug submission are shown in the Box given below:

2. The request should be sent to the DTC secretary who will arrange for the request to be formally evaluated by the responsible person – either him/herself, or drug information pharmacist, or subject expert.

Standard elements of the application form for evaluation

Generic name—List officially approved name of all chemical entities in the drug product.

Trade name—List common trade name(s) of the drug product.

Therapeutic or pharmacologic class—State the pharmaceutical or therapeutic class to which the agent belongs. Similar agents within the class may be listed.

Pharmacology—Describe the mechanism of action and related pharmacologic effects of the drug. If the mechanism is unknown, state this.

Pharmacokinetics - Describe how the drug is handled by the body. Include onset of effect, serum half-life, metabolic considerations, and route of excretion as appropriate.

Indications for use - State the indications approved for use by the Drug Control Authority. Include any additional uses under investigation.

Clinical studies - Briefly describe clinical study data supporting the indications for use. This review should be an unbiased, comparative review of studies, which identifies strengths and weaknesses as appropriate. Study description should include information about the patient population, inclusion and exclusion criteria, study design and protocol, statistical analysis, outcomes, and conclusions.

Adverse effects/warnings—List adverse effects associated with the drug and the frequency of occurrence. Describe methods to reduce or treat adverse effects. Discuss the risks and benefits of this drug therapy. Also, list any special precautions such as drug use in pregnancy and excretion of the drug into breast milk.

Drug interactions- List drug-drug and drug-food interactions associated with this agent, significance of these interactions, and methods for prevention.

Dosage range- List a dosage range for different routes of administration and indications for the drug. Include special dosing considerations for renal disease, age, and hepatic function.

Dosage form and cost- List the dosage form and strengths proposed for formulary addition. Include the cost of each dosage form and strength. A table listing comparable agents may be useful in determining the value of a formulary addition or modification.

Summary- Summarize the information provided in a single paragraph which should include

the pharmacological actions of the medicine and its proposed indication.

Is it a duplication of an existing formulary agent? If so, is it more effective? Safer? Less costly?

Why the medicine is superior to those already on the formulary list

- How should it be used?
- Who should use it?
- When should it be used?
- Are there any other special concerns?

References- Evidence from literature to support inclusion on the formulary list.

Declaration of interest - whether the applicant has received any financial support from the supplier, i.e. the manufacturing company or wholesaler.

For office use

Recommendation—State the recommendation and rationale for the recommendation. Recommended actions may include formulary addition, formulary restriction, formulary deletion, or do not add to formulary.

B. EVALUATIONS OF APPLICATIONS TO ADD NEW MEDICINES TO THE FORMULARY LIST

These should be conducted using explicit documented criteria, preferably evidence-based as previously agreed by DTC.

1. **Criteria for consideration of new treatments for conditions not amenable to existing drug therapy, or treatments representing major improvements in survival and quality of life:**

   i. The efficacy, effectiveness and safety of the medicine, as assessed by available literature.

   ii. The quality of the drug (which may be considered adequate if registered by the national regulatory body) and a supply chain of acceptable quality (with regard to manufacture, storage and transport).

   iii. Whether the hospital has the necessary clinical expertise and laboratory services to use the medicine, and what role specialists should play to regulate therapy.

   iv. An estimation of the cost (and potential savings) to the hospital should the drug be introduced – this should include costs of the medicine itself, hospitalization and investigation. For details see section on new drug assessment.

   v. Availability of the drug in the market.

2. **Criteria for treatments representing minor improvements in the therapy compared to existing listed medicines. The committee should consider all of the above and in addition:**

   i. Whether the new drug is really superior to existing ones in terms of efficacy, safety, or convenience of dosing/administration; claimed minor improvements are often proved to be unimportant.

   ii. How the total cost for a course of treatment with the new drug compares with already listed drugs.

3. **Criteria for treatments those are therapeutically equivalent to existing listed medicines. The committee should consider all the above and in addition:**

   i. Whether the new drug is really therapeutically equivalent, and not inferior, to existing drugs in terms of efficacy, safety, or convenience of dosing/administration.

   ii. Whether the total cost for a course of treatment with new medicine is less than already listed medicines.

   iii. Criteria for non-formulary medicines. If the use of non-listed drugs is allowed in certain circumstances, then these drugs need not to be included in the formulary list. Such circumstances may include:

      a. Non – response or contraindications to available medicines.

      b. Whether to continue therapy for a patient who had been stabilized on a non-listed medicine before admission to hospital and where changing to another drug is considered detrimental.

4. **Criteria for restricting the use of certain drugs to specified specialist prescribers only. Such circumstances may include:**

   i. The danger of unnecessarily increasing antimicrobial resistance with inappropriate use of third or fourth-generation antimicrobials; thus they should be limited to prescription by infectious disease or clinical microbiology specialists.

   ii. The danger of serious side effects that could occur unnecessarily even with appropriate use, for example chemotherapeutic or cytotoxic agents; thus they should be limited to prescription by specialized physicians with knowledge of these medicines.

5. **Deletion of old medicines from drug formulary**

   a. If a new medicine is added to the formulary list for reasons of improved efficacy, safety or lower price, serious consideration should be given to deleting the medicine which was previously on the formulary list for the same indication, for two reasons:

      i.   If the new medicine is better, why continue to have a less a less good "old" medicine on the list?

      ii.   If no effort is made to consider deleting medicines, none will be deleted and the formulary list will grow in size and become difficult to manage.

   b.   Routine review of different therapeutic categories is an important part of formulary management. This can be done by evaluating all the formulary medicines within each therapeutic class in a systematic way on a regular basis and comparing them to other new non- formulary medicines within that class.

   c.   A written unbiased medication review should be prepared from available literature and reviewed in the DTC meeting.

6. Written report of the drug evaluation

A written report should be compiled by the person who conducted the evaluation, and discussed at a scheduled DTC meeting. This report should contain the following information:

1. The drug monograph, including pharmacology, pharmacokinetics, efficacy compared to placebo and other medicines, clinical trial analysis, adverse drug reactions, drug interactions, cost comparison.

2. Recommendations based on the evidence-based information.

3. Expert opinion and recommendations of knowledgeable and respected physicians and pharmacists.

4. How much the new medicine would cost the hospital?

5. Whether the new drug belongs to the national/state EML and whether it is reimbursable by health insurance schemes.

7. Discussion and voting procedures

1. The report should be discussed by the DTC members and a vote taken on the recommendations presented by the person who compiled the drug evaluation report.

2. Disseminate final decision to all health-care staff in the form of minutes, in newsletters, internet and departmental meetings.

3. The committee should have established methods/rules for medication selection and review.

4. All members should declare and discuss any conflict of interests prior to discussion of the drug or drug class to make decision unbiased.

5. Document all decisions of the DTC.

V. MANAGING NON-FORMULARY DRUGS OR NON-LISTED REQUESTS

1. A register of all non-listed medicine requests (including the agent used, indications, quantity/ number of times required, alternatives available, if any, cost impact, patient safety issues) should be kept by the pharmacy along with the name of the requesting doctor.

2. When compiled at the end of the year, this list can tell the DTC about prescriber's needs and requirement or adherence to the formulary list. This information can be used for revision of the list.

VI. RESPONSIBILITIES OF A PHARMACIST

1. Participate in the DTC meetings and do follow-up with data collection, analysis and research when necessary.

2. Communicate DTC decisions to other health care professionals such as pharmacy staff, medical staff, and patient care staff.

6 | Procurement

Pharmaceutical procurement is a complex process which involves many steps, agencies, ministries, and manufacturers. Operational principles for good pharmaceutical procurement are based on four strategic objectives and are relevant to both public and private sector drug supply system which include:

1. Procure the most cost-effective drugs in the right quantities
2. Source high -quality products from reliable suppliers
3. Ensure timely delivery
4. Achieve the lowest possible total cost

For efficient procurement management unbiased market information on product availability, comparative pricing, product quality and supplier performance are required. Even if appropriate policies and procedures are in place, lack of properly trained staff in key position can doom any procurement system to failure. Often pharmacists are given this responsibility for procurement.

Major problems encountered in procurement are:

- Inadequate rules, regulations and structures
- Staff with little experience in responding to market situations
- Absence of a comprehensive procurement policy
- Insufficient funding and/or funding released irregularly especially in government
- Fragmented drug procurement at state or district level
- Lack of unbiased market information

All persons involved in store management should be fully acquainted with and participate in the procurement process and should be able to provide valuable feedback in regard to the steps involved in procurement given as below:

I. GENERAL

A written procurement policy should be available in the pharmacy. This usually assist in ensuring:

1. Product availability when required.
2. That the procurement and distribution process is fully documented.
3. That optimal storage conditions are monitored (including during transport).
4. The safety of medicines.
5. That patients receive stock that has been suitably stored and has an expiry date that allows sufficient time for usage by the patient before the expiry date.
6. That all medicines are sourced from approved suppliers only (and are therefore traceable to legitimate sources of supply).

7. Effective batch recall of medicines when necessary.

8. A store in-charge/pharmacist has a professional responsibility to exercise control over all medicinal and related products, which are purchased or supplied.

9. A purchasing policy should be in place that ensures the safety of medicine.

10. A store in-charge/pharmacist should not purchase, or supply any medicinal product where the pharmacist/dispenser has any reason to doubt its safety, quality or efficacy.

11. The store in-charge/pharmacist should know and select suppliers by applying various quality parameters, in accordance with the Drugs and Cosmetics Act and standards of Good Manufacturing Practice (GMP).

12. A store in-charge/pharmacist should be satisfied that both the supplier and the source of any medicine purchased are reputable and recorded with Drugs Control Authority. Due regard must be paid to the storage conditions before purchase and to the labels, leaflets, appearance, origin and subsequent chain of supply of the medicine concerned.

II. EFFICIENT TRANSPARENT MANAGEMENT

Procurement procedures should be transparent, following formal written procedures throughout the process and using explicit criteria to award contracts.

1. Divide procurement functions and responsibilities (selection, quantification, product specifications, pre-selection of suppliers and adjudication of tenders), among different offices, committees and individuals to ensure that no one individual is dealing with all activities and thus susceptible to undue external influences.

2. A multidisciplinary Committee (DTC) should be responsible for selection, product specifications, and review of quantification and the procurement committee for other function.

3. Procurement procedures should be transparent, following formal written procedures throughout the process and using explicit criteria to award contracts.

4. Procurement should be planned properly and procurement performance should be monitored regularly; monitoring should include an annual external audit.

III. SELECTION OF PHARMACEUTICALS

1. Public sector procurement should be limited to an essential medicines list or national/local formulary list.

2. The formulary/the Essential Medicines List using generic or International Non-Proprietary Names (INN) should be used as the basis for procurement. The DTC should decide the formulary list and approve purchase of non-formulary drugs. For details see section of Hospital Formulary.

3. Select formulary drugs carefully to ensure safety & efficacy. This includes choosing appropriate dosage forms, preparations and packaging and defining the specifications of the product to be purchased; for example, elixirs for children should not contain alcohol.

4. Order quantities should be based on a reliable estimate of actual need. For details see section on Quantification of Medical Supplies.

5. Pharmaceutical usage review programmes should be developed to ensure maximum patient benefit on the most economical basis.

IV. SUPPLIER SELECTION AND QUALITY ASSURANCE

1. Pharmaceutical products are supplied by manufacturers, wholesalers, and the local agents. Prospective suppliers should be pre-qualified, and selected suppliers should be monitored through a process, which considers product quality, service reliability, delivery time and financial viability.

2. Procure only registered products from reliable, licensed suppliers and manufacturers that comply with GMP and have good records of performance, to ensure that medicines procured meet the required standard of quality. The qualification of the suppliers can be checked by networking with other procurement agencies and Drugs Control Authority, obtaining all certification and, laboratory testing of received products. Suppliers who do not have permanent addresses or who are not prepared for visits to their premises without prior notice are unlikely to be reliable.

V. DETERMINING THE TENDER FORMAT AND GENERAL INSTRUCTIONS

Procurement methods commonly used in practice are open tender, restricted/limited tender, competitive negotiations and direct procurement depending on the total value of the tender, source, availability, etc.

1. *Bid form*: The Bidder should complete the Bid Form, which should be accompanied by the requested documentation.

2. *Language*: The Bid must be made in a national or local language or English as acceptable.

3. *Communications*: All communications must be done in same language as the Bid. Any serious communication should be done in writing by fax, e-mail, or mail and the Purchaser should respond without delay. All responses, estimated by the tender committee to be of any importance, should be sent to all prospective Bidders.

4. *Documents comprising the bid*

    The bid should comprise of the following documents:

    i. The Bid Form

    ii. A price schedule, presenting unit and total prices

    iii. Documentary evidence for Manufacturing License and Good Manufacturing Practices or World Health Organization (WHO-GMP) Certificate (if applicable).

    iv. Quality Control procedures, capacity and equipment of the Manufacturer.

    v. Documentary evidence of Quality Assurance for each item.

    vi. Incidental services and its part of the price (if applicable).

5. *Marking and mailing of bids*

    i. The bidder should seal the original and each of two copies of the bid in an inner and outer envelope, duly marking the envelopes as "original" and "copy". The outer envelope should be marked "Do not open before" plus the time and date of opening given in the bid invitation.

    ii. The inner envelope should indicate the name and address of the Bidder, to enable the bid to be returned unopened in case it is declared late.

    iii. Bids should be hand delivered or sent by courier/mail to ensure timely arrival.

    iv. If the outer envelope is not marked and sealed as required above, the Purchaser should not take any responsibility for misplacement or premature opening of the bid.

6. **Time and address for receiving bids**

   i. Bids must be received at the address no later than the date and time specified in the invitation on the front page. Any bids received after the deadline for submission of the bids should be rejected and returned unopened to the Bidder.

   ii. Bids received prior to the time of opening should be securely kept unopened.

   iii. Modifications submitted and received prior to the closing time should be considered as a part of the bid.

7. **Corrections**

   Erasures or other changes in the Bid must be explained or noted over the signature of the bidder and communicated before the day fixed for opening.

8. **Public opening of bids**

   i. Bidders or their authorized representatives may attend the public opening on the date and at the location indicated.

   ii. The Bidder's name, bid price, discounts, modifications, bid withdrawals and the presence of the requisite bid security (when applicable) and such other details as may be considered appropriate should be announced at the opening.

   iii. Minutes of the bid opening should be prepared by the purchaser and sent to each participator of the tender.

   iv. Withdrawn bids should be returned unopened to the Bidders.

9. **Errors in the Bid**

   Arithmetical errors should be rectified, without disqualifying the Bid, if the Bidder accepts the corrections. The unit price of the original Bid should be prevailing.

10. **Withdrawal of Bids**: Bids may be withdrawn on written or telegraphic request received from the Bidder prior to the time fixed for opening. Negligence on the part of the Bidder in preparing the Bid confers no right to withdrawal of the Bid after it has been opened.

11. **Rejection of Bids**

    i. The Purchaser reserves the right to reject any bid at any time during the ongoing evaluation, which does not substantially respond and conform to all terms, conditions and technical specifications of the Bidding Document.

    ii. The Purchaser reserves the right to reject any Bid, which fails to present fundamental documentation as requested in the Bidding Document and therefore appears inadequate. The Purchaser reserves the right to reject any Bid from a company previously failed to perform properly contracts of a similar nature or did not complete on time.

12. **Origin of Products**

    i. The origin of the products must be clearly stated with name, address and country of manufacture.

    ii. The country of origin must be a signatory of the agreement of the "WHO Certificate Scheme on the Quality of Pharmaceuticals Products Moving in International Commerce".

    iii. Any obscurity on the origin of products offered should disqualify the bid.

13. **Currency of Bid**: The currency of bid prices should be specified such as in Rupees or USD.

14. **Discount**: Special payment terms or other discounts should be indicated in the Bid.

15. **Validity of Bid**: Bids should be valid for a period of not less than 90 days.

16. *Delivery Terms*

   i. Bidders should quote Cost Insurance and Freight (CIF) to the indicated ports or if possible Carriage and Insurance Paid (CIP) to the indicated addresses given in the delivery schedule, as annex to the contract.

   ii. Free on Board (FOB) to a named port (including or assuming delivery without charge to a ship).

17. *Award of Contract*

   i. The determination to award the Contract to a successful Bidder should be done on a well-defined criteria laid prior to the price bid opening based on technical, quality assurance system, production, capabilities, furthermore experience and credibility of the manufacturer as well as the controlling authorities.

   ii. The Purchaser should notify the successful Bidder in writing.

VI. TECHNICAL SPECIFICATIONS AND SPECIFIC INSTRUCTIONS TO BIDDERS

1. *Quantities*: The required quantities of pharmaceuticals and medical supplies and instructions as to how the packing should be done in boxes/kits, should be specified in the "Specifications and schedule of requirements". At the time for signing a contract, there should be a possibility to negotiate with the supplier for the final quantities, independently of the initial request in the invitation.

2. *Qualifications of Manufacturers*: The Bidder should furnish copies of all certificates and documents issued by the proper national authorities, that the manufacturer of the pharmaceuticals and equipment proposed is authorized to manufacture and sell these products.

3. *Appraisal*: Placement of orders with a company, which is not known by the Purchaser or is not well recognized by the international community, would require that the company provide evidence of certification by an internationally recognized authority (e.g. FDA or similar, as approved by the Purchaser) or be subject, at the Company's expense, to inspection by a competent authority designated by the Purchaser in conjunction with the national regulatory authority.

4. *Standards and quality assurance for supply*

   i. Any pharmaceutical product offered must be manufactured in conformity with the latest edition of Indian, British, International, United States, French or European Pharmacopoeia. If the product is not included in the specified Compendia, the Bidder upon being awarded the order, must provide the reference standards and testing protocols to allow for Quality Control.

   ii. Any offered product must be manufactured in accordance with Good Manufacturing Practices (GMP) standards established by the World Health Organization or Schedule M as given in Drugs & Cosmetics Act (Appendix 1).

   iii. All pharmaceutical products must:

      a. meet the requirements of manufacturing legislation and regulation of pharmaceuticals and medicines

      b. authority in the manufacturer's country according to resolution WHA 28.65B and WHA 41.18 of the World Health Organization "WHO Certification Scheme on the Quality of Pharmaceuticals Products Moving in International Commerce" (which can be obtained in WHO Headquarters or from the WHO Country Representative).

iv.   indicate the dates of manufacture and expiry.

v.   Arrive at the port of entry (for imported pharmaceuticals) or warehouse (for local purchases) with a remaining shelf life of at least 75% of the total stipulated shelf life at the time of manufacture.

vi.   On request, make available samples and studies showing bioavailability and stability, especially stability under conditions of high temperature and humidity.

vii.   Prove the quality of packing and the appearance of labels through representative samples on request.

5.   *Product Information*

The following information is required, when applicable, for each product offered by the Bidder:

i.   Generic name or INN (International Non-proprietary Name)

ii.   Presentation, strength, quantity in each container

iii.   Country of origin, name and address of the Manufacturer

iv.   Pharmacopoeia or other applicable compendia standards

v.   Proper documentation of quality assurance.

vi.   Shelf life

vii.   Type of container

Failure to include any of this information may at the discretion of the purchaser, disqualify the bid.

6.   *Labelling*: The language of the labels should be as per requirement in the bid document (English/vernacular).

The label for each pharmaceutical product should meet the GMP standard and include:

i.   The INN or generic name prominently displayed

ii.   The active ingredient per unit, dose, tablet or capsule, etc. (strength & presentation)

iii.   The applicable pharmacopoeia standard

iv.   The Purchaser's logo and code number, if required

v.   Content per container

vi.   Instructions for use (only on instructions by the purchaser)

vii.   Special storage requirements

viii.   Batch number

ix.   Date of manufacture and date of expiry

x.   Name and address of Manufacturer

xi.   Country of origin

xii.   "keep out of reach of children"

xiii.   The outer carton should also display the above information.

7.   *Pharmaceutical packing*

i.   Containers for Pharmaceuticals must conform with any of the latest of the internationally recognized Pharmacopoeia Standards, such as Indian, British, United States or European.

ii.   The size of the container should be proportional to its content, with the additional appropriate padding to prevent damage to the product during transport.

   iii. Containers should be tamper-proof.

   iv. Ampoules should be one ended and autobreakable

8. *Packing of Goods*.

The Vendor should ensure that the packing of goods is according to appropriate commercial standards and adequate to protect the goods for carriage by sea to the agreed port of entry or address of delivery.

VII. CONDITIONS OF CONTRACT

1. *Language* - The language of the contract should be national or vernacular or English.

2. *Indemnification*

   i. The Vendor should indemnify and protect the purchaser against claims, damages, losses, costs and expenses arising out of any injury, sickness or death to persons or any loss of or damage to property, caused by the fault or negligence of the Vendor. The Vendor warrants that the goods offered for sale under the contract do not infringe any patent, trade-name, or trade-mark. In addition, the Vendor should indemnify, defend and protect the Purchaser from any actions or claims brought against the Purchaser pertaining to alleged infringements of a patent, design, tradesman or trade-mark arising from the contract.

   ii. Any export licenses or other licences required for the goods should be obtained by the Vendor.

   iii. Any levies imposed on the goods outside the Purchaser's country, should be the entire responsibility of the Supplier.

3. *Performance Security*

   i. Within 30 days after the Supplier's receipt of notification of award of the Contract, the Supplier should furnish performance security to the Purchaser such as in the amount of 10% of the Contract Price.

   ii. The proceeds of the performance security should be payable to the Purchaser as compensation for any loss resulting from the Supplier's failure to complete his obligations under the Contract.

   iii. The Performance Security should be paid in a manner agreed on and accepted by the Purchaser.

   iv. The performance security should be discharged by the Purchaser and returned to the Supplier not later than four (4) months following the date of final delivery to the destinations indicated to the Contract.

4. *Inspections and Tests*

   i. The purchaser or its representative should have full access to the facilities of the supplier at all reasonable times to appraise the production, testing and packaging of the material, and should provide reasonable assistance to the Purchaser or its representative for such appraisal. That may includes also copies of any relevant test results or Quality Control protocols that may be necessary.

   ii. Should any inspected or tested Goods fail to conform to the Technical Specifications, the Purchaser may reject them and the Supplier should either replace the rejected goods or make all alterations necessary to meet the specified requirements free of cost to the Purchaser.

5. *Transportation and delivery*

   i.   The goods supplied under the contract should be delivered "CIF" or "CIP" as defined in the current edition of the International Rules for the Interpretation of the Trade Terms.

   ii. Delivery of the contracted goods should be made to the ports or addresses as specified in the contract by the Purchaser.

6. *Warranty*

   i.   The Supplier warrants that all Goods supplied under the contract should fully comply in all respects with the technical specifications and with the conditions laid down in the Contract. In the event any of the Goods are recalled, the Supplier should notify the Purchaser within fourteen (14) days and promptly replace the items covered by the recall at its own cost.

   ii. If any item fails to comply with the technical specifications the supplier should promptly with all reasonable speed replace the item without cost to the Purchaser.

   iii. The Purchaser should have the right to make claims under the above warranty for the entire period of specified shelf life of each item respectively.

7. *Documentation on Delivery*

   Immediately on shipment of the contracted Goods, the Supplier should advise the Purchaser by email, fax, etc. of the following details:

   i.   Name of the vessel or carrier

   ii. Date and time of departure from port of shipment

   iii. Quantity of goods on board

   iv. Invoiced value of the Goods

   v.   Bills of lading[12] number(s)

   vi. Expected time of arrival at port of discharge

   vii. The Supplier should also dispatch to the Purchaser one set of the following documents by courier service and another set through the Master of the vessel:

      a. One negotiable copy of the clean bill of lading with non-negotiable copies (marked "freight prepaid" in CIF Contracts).

      b. Certified commercial invoice and ten copies.

      c. Original copy of the packing list.

      d. Original copy of the certificate of inspection furnished to Supplier by the nominated inspection agency and six copies.

      e. Certificate of in-house analysis.

      f. Original copy of the certificate of weight issued by the port authority/licensed authority and ten copies.

      g. Insurance Certificate.

      h. Supplier's/manufacturer's warrantee.

      i. Copy of email/fax sent to Purchaser by Supplier upon the departure of the vessel.

---

12 Lading is the action of loading a ship with cargo. Bill of lading is a legal document issued by a carrier to a Shipper detailing the details of the type, quantity and destination of the goods.

8. *Payment*

   Payment should be made in the following manner:

   i.   On shipment: 90% of the Contract Price of the Goods shipped should be paid through irrevocable confirmed Letter of Credit established in favour of the Supplier in a bank indicated by the Supplier, on submission of documents specified or any way of payment agreed on between the Supplier and the Purchaser; and

   ii. On Receipt of Goods: 10% of the Contract Price of Goods received should be paid within 30 days of receipt of Goods on submission of an invoice supported by documentary evidence issued by the Purchaser's representative that the Goods have been received.

   iii. Any other agreement on payment performance, made between the Purchaser and the Supplier will , when clearly expressed in the contract, overrule this paragraph.

   iv. The Supplier's requests(s) for payment should be made to the Purchaser in writing, accompanied by an invoice describing, as appropriate, the Goods delivered and Services performed, and by shipping documents, submitted pursuant and upon fulfillment of other obligations stipulated in the Contract.

   v.   Payments should be made promptly by the Purchaser within sixty (60) days of submission of an invoice by the Supplier.

9. *Price and Currency*.

   i.   Prices charged by the Supplier for Goods delivered and Services performed under the Contract should not vary from the prices quoted by the Supplier in its bid.

   ii. The currency of payment.

10. *Delays*

    i.   Delivery of the goods and performance of services should be made by the supplier in accordance with the time schedule specified by the purchaser in its schedule of Requirements.

    ii. An unexcused delay by the Supplier in the performance of its delivery obligations should render the Supplier liable to any or all of the following sanctions: forfeiture of its performance security, imposition of liquidated damages, and/or termination of the contract for default.

    iii. If at any time during performance of the contract, the Supplier or its subcontractor(s) should encounter conditions impeding timely delivery of the Goods and performance of Services, the Supplier should promptly notify the Purchaser in writing of the fact of the delay, it's likely duration and its cause(s). As soon as possible after receipt of the Supplier's notice, the Purchaser should evaluate the situation and may at its discretion extend the Supplier's time for performance, in which case the extension should be ratified by the parties by amendment of the Contract.

11. *Liquidated Damages*

    If the Supplier fails to deliver any or all of the Goods or perform the Services within the time period(s) specified in Specifications and Schedule of Requirements, the Purchaser should, without prejudice to its other corrective measures under the Contract, deduct from the Contract Price, as liquidated damages, a sum equivalent to 0.5% of the delivered Contract Price of the delayed Goods or unperformed Services for each week of delay until actual delivery or performance, up to a maximum deduction of 10% of the delayed Goods or Services Contract Price. Once the maximum is reached, the Purchaser may consider termination of the Contract.

12. *Termination for Default*

The Purchaser may, without prejudice to any other corrective measures for breach of contract, by written notice of default sent to the Supplier, terminate the Contract in whole or in part:

i. If the Supplier fails to deliver any or all of the Goods within the time period(s) specified in the Contract, or any extension thereof granted by the Purchaser.

ii. If the Supplier fails to replace promptly any Goods rejected when submitted for testing or subject to a recall ordered by the applicable regulatory authority in the country of manufacture due to unacceptable quality or reports of adverse drug reactions after giving prompt notice of the recall;

iii. If the Supplier fails to perform any other obligations(s) under the Contract. In the event that the Purchaser terminates the Contract in whole or in part, pursuant to paragraph above, the Purchaser may procure, upon such terms and in such manner as it deems appropriate, Goods similar to those undelivered, and the Supplier should be liable to the Purchaser for any excess costs for such similar Goods. If the Supplier fails to reimburse the Purchaser for such excess costs within a reasonable period, the Purchaser may have recourse.

13. *Force Majeure*[13]

The supplier should not be liable for forfeiture of its performance security, liquidated damages or termination for default if the delay in performance or other failure to perform its obligation under the contract is the result of an event of Force majeure. If a force majeure situation arises, the Supplier should promptly notify the Purchase in writing of such a condition and the cause thereof.

14. *Resolution of Disputes*

The Purchase and the Supplier should make every effort to resolve amicably by direct informal negotiation any disagreement or dispute arising between them under or in connection with the contract. If contract disputes is not resolved amicably by informal negotiation, the either party may require that the dispute be referred for resolution to the formal mechanism for adjudication/arbitration in accordance with the laws of the Purchaser's country or in case of international/foreign supplier the dispute should be settled by arbitration in accordance with the provisions of the UNCITRAL Model Law on Arbitration Rules.

VIII. FINANCING AND COMPETITION

1. Mechanisms should be put in place to ensure reliable financing for procurement. Good financial management procedures should be followed to maximize the use of financial resources.

2. Procurement should be effected in the largest possible quantities in order to achieve economies of scale; this applies to both centralized and decentralized systems.

3. Procurement in the public health sector should be based on competitive procurement methods, except for very small or emergency orders.

4. Members of the purchasing groups should purchase all contracted items from the supplier(s) which hold(s) the contract.

---

13 'Force Majeure" means an event beyond the control of the Supplier, not involving the Supplier's fault or negligence and not foreseeable. Such events may include but are not restricted to , acts of the Purchaser in its sovereign capacity, wars or revolutions, fires, floods, epidemics, quarantine restrictions and freight embargoes.

5. Buy in bulk, if possible to get value for money by either central rate contract or DTCs of small hospitals can collaborate with other hospitals.

6. Procurement in the public sector should be based on competitive procurement methods, except for very small or emergency orders.

7. Agree on a regular procurement schedule and decide criteria for emergency purchase in circumstances where it is absolutely indispensable to prevent immediate danger of life.

8. Purchase only from the manufacturers and their authorized representatives who holds the current contract as decided through the competitive tender adjudication process to ensure the lowest possible purchase price.

9. *Supplier Selection and Quality Assurance:* Prospective suppliers should be pre-qualified, and selected suppliers should be monitored through a process, which considers product quality, service reliability, delivery time and financial viability.

10. Procurement procedures/systems should include all assurances that the drugs purchased are of high quality, according to international standards.

IX. SUPPLY ORDER

1. The onus is on the supplier or distributor to ensure that all legal requirements are met, when medicines or scheduled substances are supplied.

2. Suppliers and distributors should ensure that accounts are only opened or agreements entered for purposes of the sale of medicines and scheduled substances in the name of the legal entity (company, close corporation, partnership or sole proprietor), which is appropriately authorized to purchase such medicine.

3. The contract should specify the penalties for default.

4. Only accept medicines with the appropriate documentation including:

    i. A certificate of analysis issued by the manufacturer (Batch certificate)

    ii. Detailed product specifications including quality standards (IP, BP., USP), labeling, nomenclature, and packaging.

    iii. For imported medicines, a WHO- GMP certificate issued by the drug regulatory authorities of the exporting country.

5. Ensure quality through the inclusion of pre-tendering criteria, for example specifying a minimum shelf life (at least 75% shelf life should remain upon arrival), and insisting manufacturers have a minimum turnover for the product quoted and proof of GMP compliance.

X. PLACING AN ORDER

1. Place your order using an order form. Some health facilities use requisition forms or books for ordering supplies from district or national stores. Each order is numbered sequentially. Pre-printed requisition forms make ordering easier and help to avoid mistakes.

2. When placing an order or re-ordering:

    i. Check the stock records to find out the stock balance and decide what items and how much of each item you need to order.

    ii. List the supplies to be ordered alphabetically and in sections, for example, drugs, equipment, consumables. Only include one item and one item size on each line. If you are ordering from a catalogue, write down the catalogue code number for each item.

iii. Provide a full and clear description of each item.

iv. Specify the quantity of each item. Place orders for complete packs. For example, if you need 34 rolls of crepe bandage and a pack contains 12 rolls, order 3 packs.

v. Check that all copies of the order are easy to read and signed by an authorised person.

vi. Check that the order includes your full contact details and, if you are not the recipient, include the contact details of the person, agency or institution to which the goods should be delivered.

vii. Make at least two copies of the order. Keep one copy in the health facility and send one copy to the supplier.

viii. Specify, if appropriate, whether the item is to be delivered or collected, the method of shipment (for example, sea, land or air), contact details of the organisations responsible for shipment and payment, and instructions for packing (for example, carton size and weight).

ix. Include any other special instructions (for example, no delivery at weekends or during holidays) and, if applicable, account number.

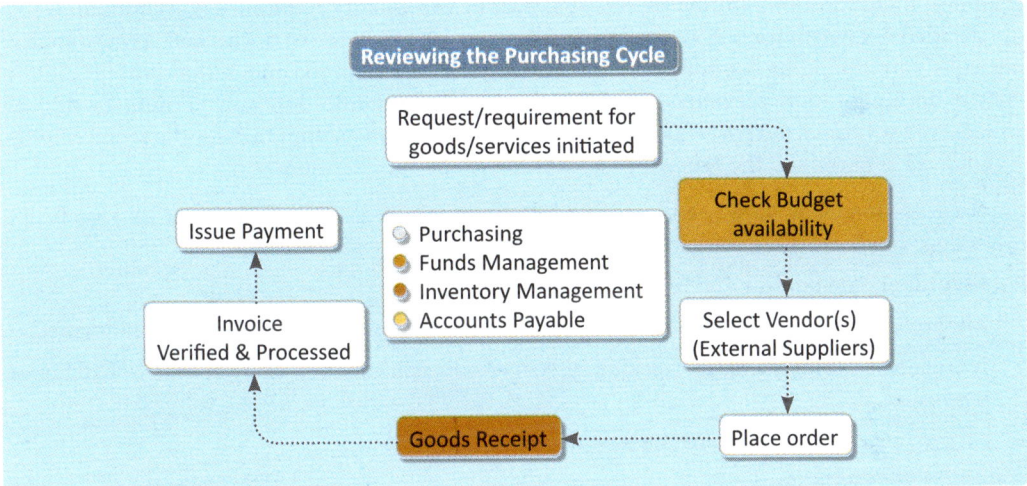

XI. PURCHASES AND ISSUE

1. Records should be kept of each purchase and sale, showing the following:

   i. Date of purchase or supply;

   ii. Name of the medicine or scheduled substance;

   iii. Quantity received or supplied;

   iv. Name and address of the supplier or consignee;

   v. Batch number and expiry date.

2. A valid written order must be obtained prior to any sale and/or dispatch of specified Schedule X item. This order, as well as record keeping of all sales of specified Schedule X must comply with legislative requirements.

3. Records should ensure the traceability of the origin and destination of products, for example by use of batch numbers, so that all the suppliers of, or those supplied with a medicine or scheduled substance can be identified.

4. Manual/computerized, list of documents to be maintained along with Invoice bin card, Stock card/Stock Ledger/Kardex forms.

XII. ISSUING SUPPLIES

1. Every health facility also needs a system for recording issue of supplies. The most common method is an issue book or issue voucher (see Appendix 2).

2. The following information should be recorded every time an item is issued:

    i.   Date of issue, item and quantities issued,

    ii. Name of receiving service or individual, and the signature of the recipient.

3. Give a copy of the issue voucher to the recipient for their records.

4. After issue, the receiving service or individual should be responsible for care of the item and accountable for loss or breakage. For example, microscope care should be the responsibility of the laboratory or the laboratory technician in-charge.

XIII. DOCUMENTATION, RECORDKEEPING AND ACCOUNTING

Good documentation constitutes an essential part of the Quality Assurance (QA) system. Good and detailed documentation is an essential obligation for discharge of duties and accountability. Particular care should be taken to ensure that all events are recorded and authenticated. Clearly written documentation prevents errors from spoken communication and permits tracing of procedures for various purposes. Documents should be detailed enough to meet the requirements of audit and in particular the following should receive special attention:

1. Records should be made at the time of each operation in such a way that all significant activities or events are traceable.

2. Records should be clear and readily available.

3. All records must be retained for the legislative period applicable for the product concerned.

4. It is useful to employ a batch-tracking system which enables the tracking of specific batches of medicines.

5. All product complaints should be duly noted.

7 Supply Chain Management and Distribution of Pharmaceuticals

I. MANAGING SUPPLY CHAIN

The primary management goal is to maintain a steady supply of drugs and supplies to facilities where they are needed in good condition while ensuring that resources are being used in the most effective way. A well run distribution system should:

1. Maintain a constant supply of drug
2. Keep drugs in good condition
3. Minimize drug losses due to spoilage and expiry
4. Use available transport as efficiently as possible
5. Reduce theft & pilferage
6. Provide information for forecasting of drug needs

A. DISTRIBUTION CYCLE

The distribution cycle begins when drugs are dispatched by the manufacturer or supplier. It ends when drug consumption information is reported back to the procurement unit. The major activities of the distribution cycle include:

1. Quarantine incoming goods
2. Check documents by inspection teams
3. Check sample for quality assurance
4. Inspection by inspection team
5. Reporting
6. Release into stock
7. Consumption reporting

B. DISTRIBUTION SEQUENCE

Drug procurement: The distribution sequence intersects the procurement process at the point at which drugs are available for delivery to the health facilities.

Receipt and inspection: Conduct complete inspection of every shipment as soon as it is received from the port or local supplier. The shipment must be kept separate from other stock until this inspection has been completed. Inspectors should check for damaged and missing items and for compliance with the contract conditions concerning drug type, quantity, presentation, packaging, labeling and any special requirements. Prompt and accurate inspection of all shipments is essential to ensure that suppliers fulfill their contracts.

Inventory control: Establishing and maintaining effective inventory records and procedures are the basis for coordinating the flow of drugs through the distribution system and the primary protection against theft and corruption. The inventory control system is used for requisitioning and issuing drugs, for financial accounting, and for preparing the consumption and stock balance reports necessary for procurement. Record keeping must be sufficiently detailed to provide and "audit trail" that accurately traces the flow of drugs and funds through the system. This audit trail must be designed to satisfy the requirements of government auditors (and sometimes donor agencies) as well as programme managers.

An appropriate inventory management system should be adapted to suit the capacity and needs of personnel at all levels in the health programme. Inventory records must be monitored regularly by supervisors to ensure accuracy and to avoid losses. For details see section on Inventory Management and Quantification of Medical Supplies.

Storage: Storage facilities may range from large mechanized warehouses at the national level to small wooden boxes sitting in health centers or carried by community health workers. Proper location, construction, organization and maintenance of storage facilities help maintain drug quality, minimize theft and maintain regular supply to health facilities.

Requisition of Supplies: Drug supply systems may operate under a push or a pull system. The form and procedures for requisition are a key part of the inventory control system. They may vary from country to country and from one level to another within the same country. The requisition system may be manual or computerized, but it should always be designed to simplify distribution by facilitating inventory control, providing an adult trial for tracing the flow of drugs, assisting in financial accounting, and listing drugs issued.

Delivery: Drugs may be delivered by warehouses or collected by health facilities. Transport may involve, air, water, railway, or on and off-road vehicles. Cost effective choices between public and private sector carriers need to be made. Transport managers should select methods of transportation carefully and schedule deliveries realistically and systematically to provide punctual and economic service. Vehicle breakdowns, availability of fuel, lubricants, and spare parts; seasonal variation in access routes; safety along specific supply lines; and other local factors must all be considered in transport planning.

Dispensing to patients: The distribution process achieves its purpose when drugs reach hospital wards, outpatient clinics, health centers or community health workers and are appropriately prescribed and dispensed to patients.

Consumption Reporting: The closing link in the distribution cycle is the flow of information on consumption and stock balances back up distribution system to procurement office for use in quantifying procurement needs. If adequate inventory and requisition records are kept, compiling consumption reports should be straightforward.

II. EVALUATING THE EXISTING SYSTEM

The first step involved in improving the logistics of drug supply is to analyze the existing system against the checklist set out below:

A. DISTRIBUTION NETWORK

1. How is the distribution network organized?
    i. Where are the major supply sources located?
    ii. Where are the storage facilities located?
    iii. Where are the clinical facilities located?

iv. How many levels does the distribution hierarchy have?

v. What are the transport routes between facilities?

vi. What means of transport are used?

2. How is the distribution system administered?

3. What are travel times and mileages between warehouses and clinical facilities?

4. Are there significant regional variations in travel times and mileages?

5. How much are travel times affected by seasonal factors (rainy, winter seasons, etc.)?

B. STORAGE (EACH FACILITY)

1. How is the storage facility organized?

   i. Staff organization chart?

   ii. Physical layout of storage and administrative facilities?

   iii. Stock administration procedures?

   iv. Transport organization?

   v. Building maintenance arrangements?

   vi. Transport and equipment maintenance arrangements?

2. How well do the basic routines of receiving, storage and shipping work?

3. At central level only: From date of dispatch by the supplier(s), how long does it take for drugs to arrive at the central medical store(s) and from central medical stores to the district and health facility?

4. How long does it take to process a requisition and prepare a shipment?

5. How long does it take to determine the quantity of each item in stock?

6. Using the VED categories (Vital, Essential and Desirable drugs), how many vital, essential and desirable drug items have been out-of-stock in the previous 12 months, and for how long?

7. What is the physical condition of:

   i. The pharmaceutical stock?

   ii. The buildings?

   iii. Air conditioning and refrigeration equipment?

   iv. The handling equipment?

   v. The transport fleet?

8. Is the size of the building correct?

III. DESIGNING A DISTRIBUTION AND STORAGE SYSTEM

The steps involved in designing or modifying a distribution system are as follows:

A. ESTABLISH A DISTRIBUTION NETWORK

1. Determine the optimum number of levels in the distribution network and the delivery routes between the facilities. Work towards a system that is simple to manage and which keeps costs as low as possible whilst providing regular, scheduled drug deliveries that minimize the risk of stock outs.

2. Factors which influence distribution network design are:

   i. Number and geographical distribution of clinical facilities.

ii. Effect of route and distance on the time taken to reach these facilities.

iii. Number, type and capacity of existing storage facilities.

iv. Management skills at each level.

v. Transport alternatives, their relative costs and their dependability. A basic requirement of system design is to establish the number of levels in the distribution hierarchy. This is a complex process.

3. Direct delivery models are generally less expensive to set up, to operate and to manage. However, where travel times and geographical separation are great, Central Medical Store (CMS) systems often provide a better service. They may even be cheaper to operate since they may reduce the need to airlift supplies during adverse weather or epidemics.

4. Make a diagram of the existing distribution network, including all clinical and storage facilities and their supply lines. Establish the network throughout at each node in the network and estimate current inventory costs.

5. Make a diagram of up to six feasible alternative networks. Include patterns based on different linkages between existing facilities as well as once that require new facilities.

6. For each alternative, estimate as accurately as possible the costs and benefits associated with the system characteristics. Establish the network throughout of the drugs needed at each node in alternative distribution networks and assess whether this can be achieved. Estimate inventory costs for each alternative.

7. Select and implement the system that provides the best quality of service with available funds, or justify and make application for additional funds, or justify additional funds based on arguments of improved effectiveness.

8. Some delivery models are shown below:

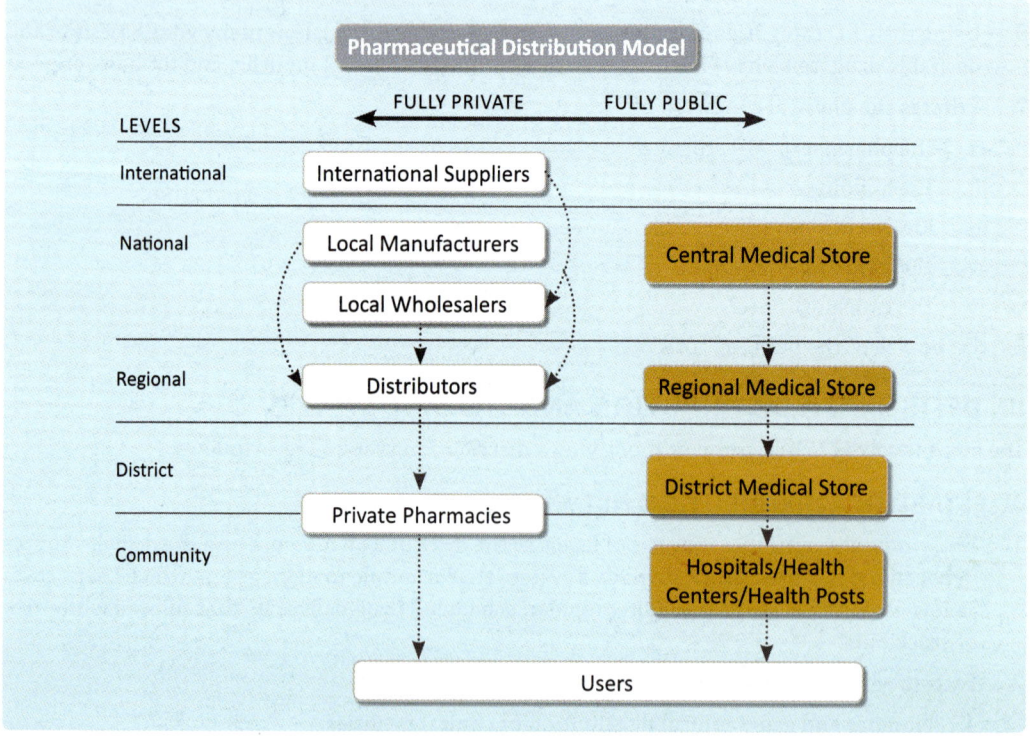

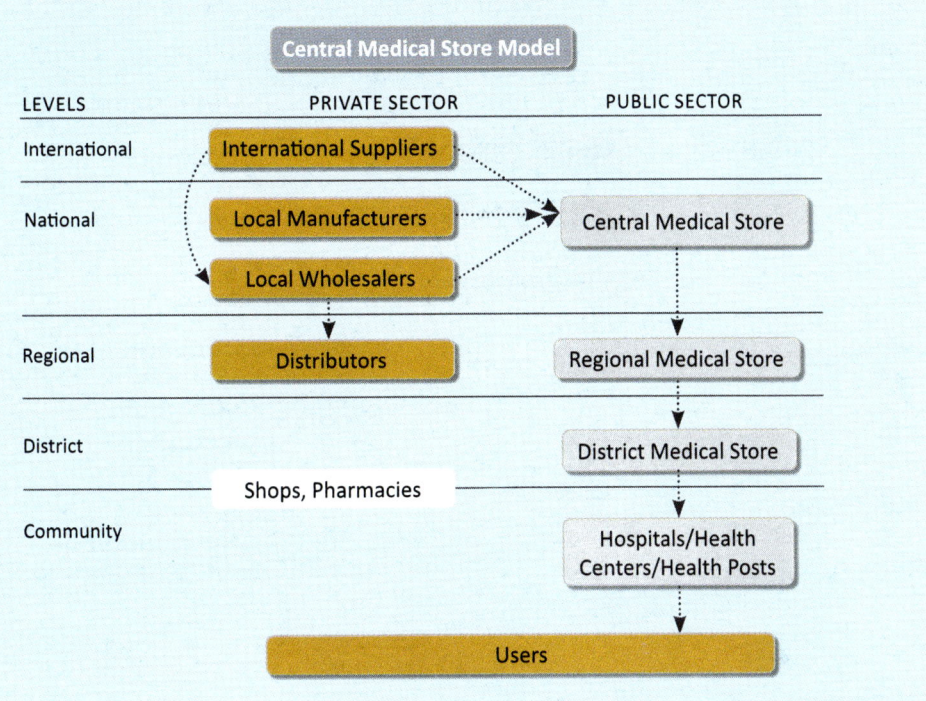

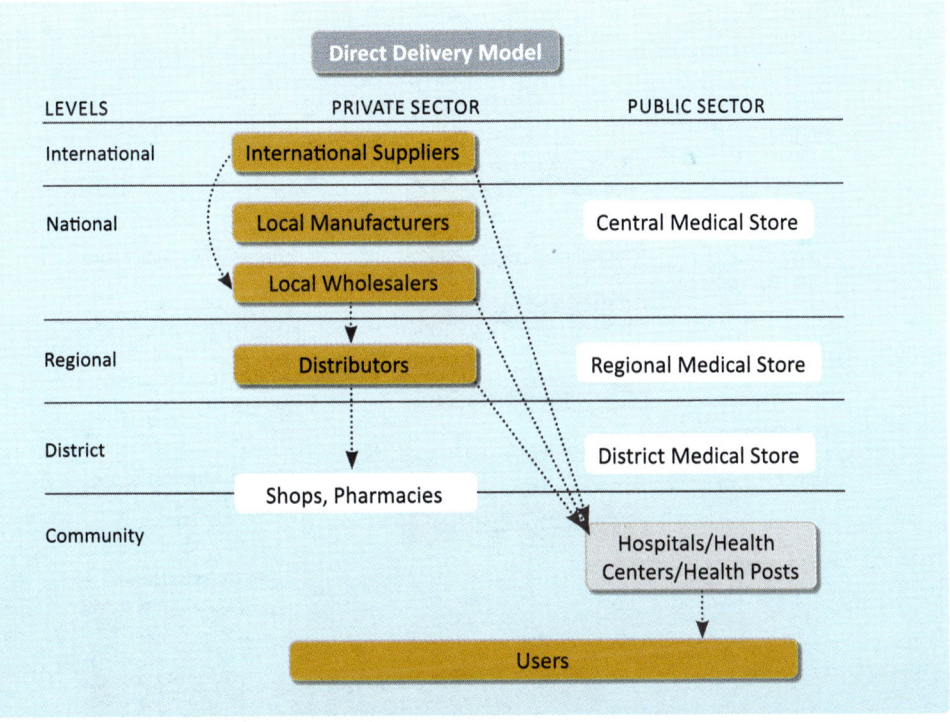

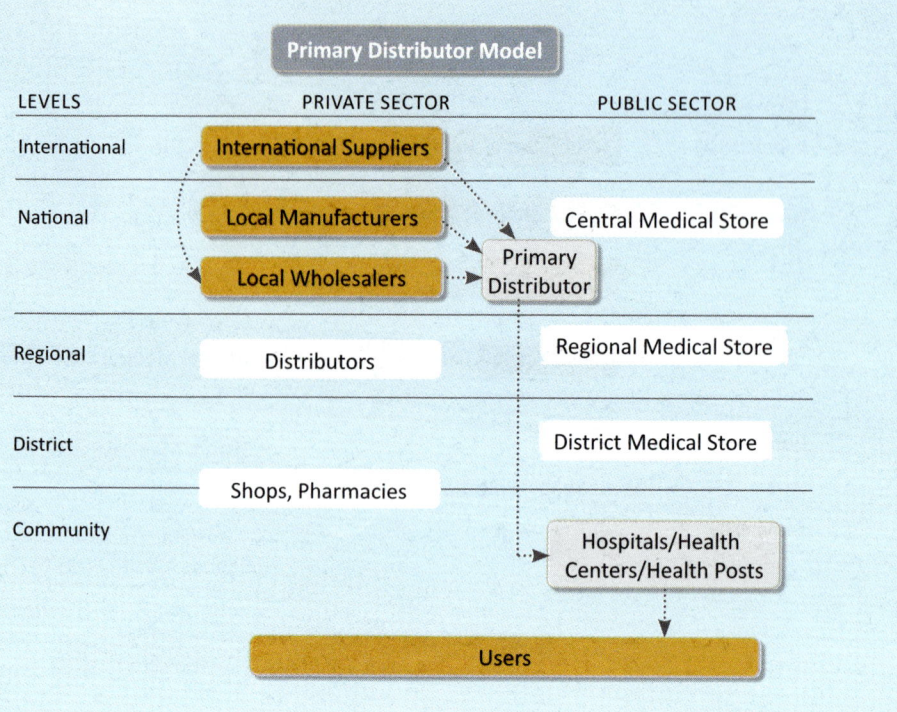

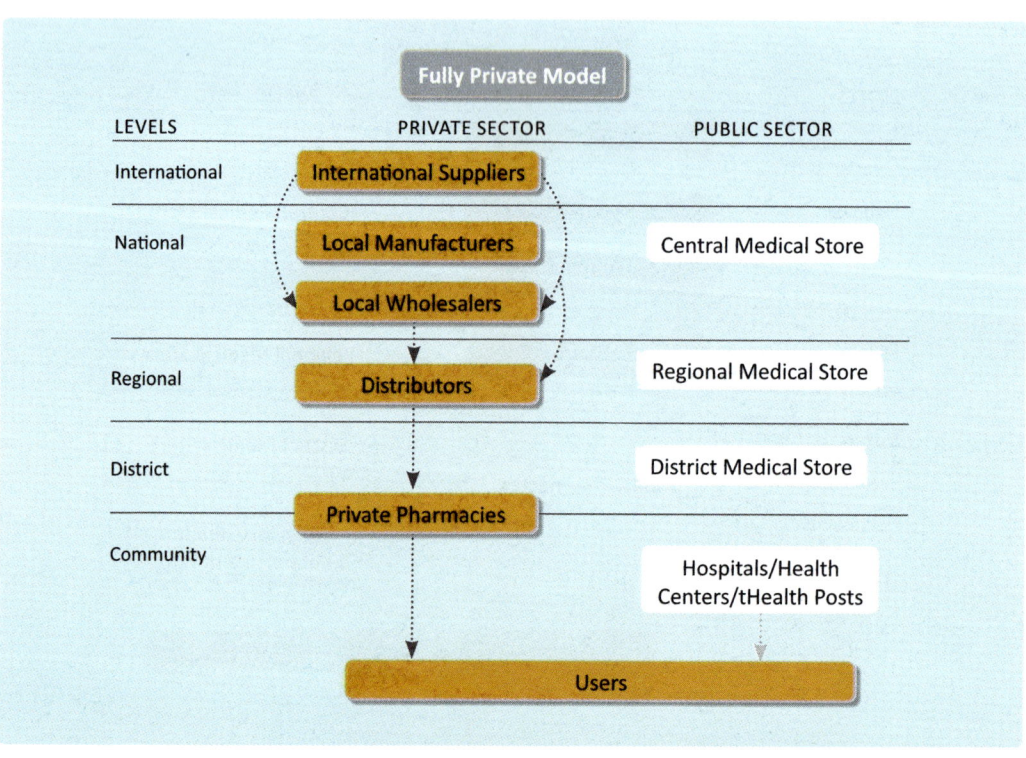

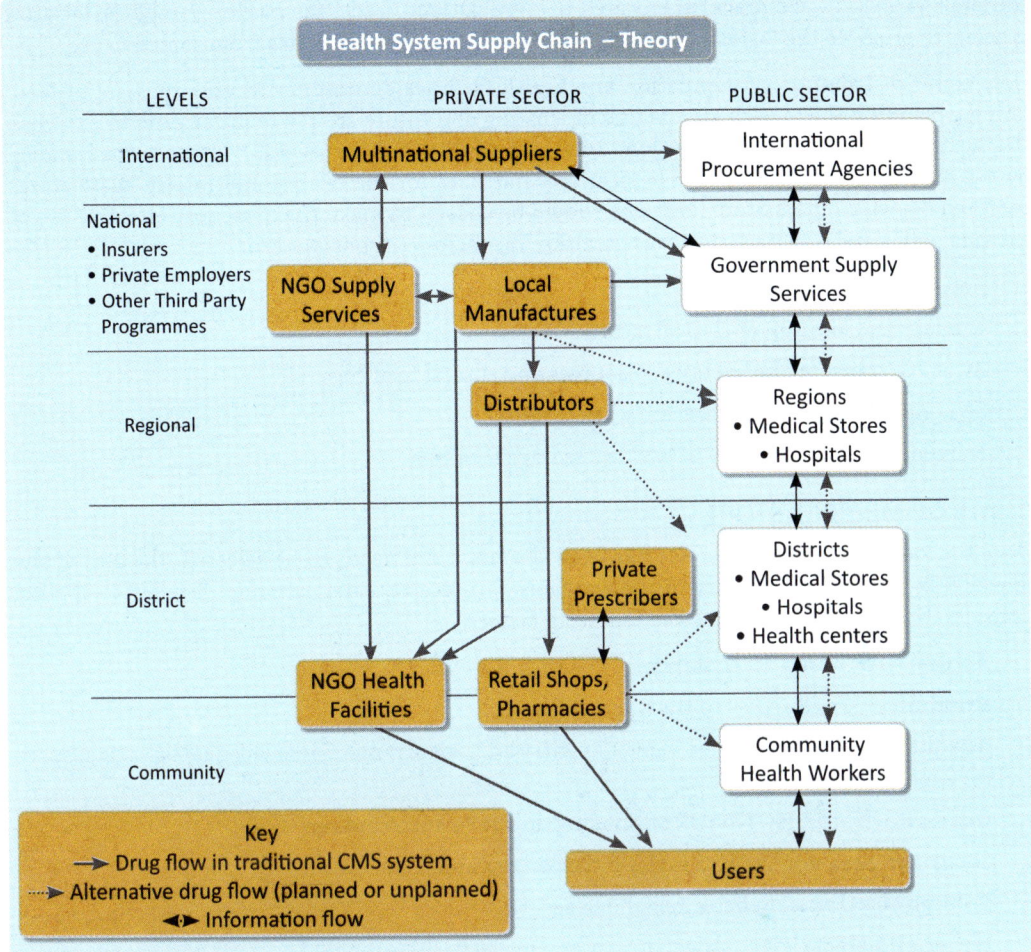

9. Whichever distribution channel is used all parties involved in the distribution of pharmaceutical products should be identified. All parties have a responsibility to ensure that the quality of pharmaceutical products and the integrity of the distribution chain is maintained throughout the distribution process from the site of the manufacturer to the entity responsible for dispensing or providing the product to the patient.

10. Measures should be in place to ensure that pharmaceutical products have documentation (including expiry date, batch number) that can be used to permit traceability of the products throughout distribution channels from the manufacturer/importer to the entity responsible for selling or supplying the product to the patient.

11. Good storage practices (GSP) are applicable in all circumstances where pharmaceutical products are stored and throughout the distribution process. For additional guidance relating to the general principles of storage of pharmaceutical products, see chapter on Medical Store Management.

B. LOCATION OF THE MEDICAL STORE

The placement of medical stores can be described in terms of location and site. Location refers to the city, town or geographical position of the warehouse. Whilst clinical facilities (which may contain pharmaceutial storage) are located to serve patient needs, the goal of warehouse location is solely to promote the fastest and least expensive transport of supplies from source to user.

Geographic distribution of population and health facilities determines where drugs are needed. Storage planning starts with an analysis of existing and future supply requirements to establish the type and quantity of drugs required by each facility and the overall volume to be handled by the distribution system. Suitable locations and sizes for the central and intermediate stores can then be determined. Store locations should be chosen to make the most cost-effective use of existing public and private transport networks. The factors to consider are:

1. Location of supply sources.
2. Number and location of clinical facilities.
3. Available transport links between sources and clinical facilities.
4. Seasonal factors that may severely affect routes.
5. Number, type and capacity of existing storage facilities.

C. SITE OF MEDICAL STORES

Once the location of the warehouse has been chosen, a site needs to be selected. The aim of site selection is to ensure the ability of the warehouse to receive, safeguard and distribute supplies. Consideration should be given to the following factors:

1. **Access:** Year round accessibility.
2. **Proximity:** Good access to transport links.
3. **Adequate size:** Unimpaired vehicular entry and exit arrangements, adequate parking, space for expansion.
4. **Good site drainage:** No risk of flooding on site or surroundings.
5. **Security:** Area not likely to invite intrusion or vandalism.
6. **Communications:** Reliable telephone service.
7. **Water and electricity:** Adequate water and electricity supply.
8. **Housing:** Adequate housing, etc., available for staff within reach or warehouse.

D. PUSH AND PULL SYSTEMS

An essential decision must be made as to which levels of the system will order drugs and which, if any, will passively receive drugs distributed from higher levels. The two basic alternatives are:

1. **Pull system:** Each level of the system determines what types and quantities of drugs are needed and places orders with the supply source (which may be a warehouse in the system or a commercial supplier). This type of system is sometimes called an independent demand or a requisition system.
2. **Push system:** Supply sources at some level in the system determine what types and quantities of drugs will be delivered to lower levels. A delivery plan is made at the beginning of a planning period, usually a year, and supplies are delivered according to the plan. This is also known as an allocation or a ration system the best known example in drug supply is the ration kit system.

When using a pull system, managers of operations units are expected to work out their own demand estimates and buffer stocks and submit requisitions to central stores indicating their requirements. In a push system, operational units are expected to supply certain stock and consumption information to the supply source so that issuing officers can plan allocation.

Pull systems are preferred whenever the capacity exists to manage them effectively. However, there are situation in which a push system is useful, such as disaster relief and when the supply pipeline does not function at all level of the system. Conditions that tend to favor push and pull distribution systems are presented below:

Conditions Favouring a Pull System

1. Lower-level staff is competent in assessing needs and managing inventory.
2. Sufficient supplies are available at supply sources to meet all programme needs.
3. A large range of products is being handled.
4. Field staffs are regularly supervised, and performance is monitored.

Condition Favouring a Push System

1. Lower-level staff are not competent in inventory control.
2. Demand greatly exceeds supply, making rationing necessary.
3. A limited number of products is being handled.
4. Disaster relief is needed, or the situation calls for short term supply through prepared kits.

Re-supply interval

Once the choice between a push and a pull system has been made, the next step is to select an appropriate re-supply interval. This determines whether deliveries are made to user units quarterly, monthly, weekly, or at any other time. If deliveries are made weekly, average stock levels will be low and the likelihood of stock outs will decrease, but transport costs will be very high. If deliveries are made only once a year, transport costs will be low but the average stocks and storage costs will be high.

The optimum re-supply interval needs to be worked out to suit individual programme needs. Most public programmes use intervals of one to three months. It is helpful to consider the following factors before making a decision:

1. Storage capacity at each level of the system
2. Availability, order size, carrying capacity and cost of transport
3. Seasonal factors that influence transport reliability
4. Staffing levels and competence of staff at each level of the system.
5. Other factors, such as expiration dates, security against pilferage, and other locally relevant concerns.

Storage Capacity

The capacity of each existing store should be assessed. If the existing storage capacity is insufficient, five possible solutions are available:

1. Reorganize the store by changing the shelving layout or by introducing pallet racking
2. Build or rent additional warehouse space. This option involves capital costs for warehouse construction or recurrent costs for warehouse rental.
3. Increase the supply frequency to eliminate the need for additional storage space, probably at some increase in administrative costs. Suppliers may also charge extra for more frequent delivery. If the supply interval is already short, it may not be practical to decrease it.
4. Upgrade another underutilized lower-level stores to higher level status.

5. If insufficient space at the primary level is the problem, consider holding larger stocks at the intermediate level, assuming the capacity exists.

6. A system based on regular transfer of stock between stores at the same level should be avoided in most cases, because it is difficult to record such movements. However, some supply systems can manage redistribution, depending on the qualifications and motivation of the personnel involved.

Delivery Systems versus Collection System

The next important decision to be made concerns how supplies will be moved between the warehouse and the receiving facility. Basically there are two options: collection or delivery. In the case of a collection system, the receiving facility takes on the responsibility for collecting supplies from the warehouse. In a delivery system the warehouse is responsible for delivering supplies with either in-house transport or a private sector contract.

Each method has advantages and disadvantages; the choice should be based on individual programme needs and constraints. General advantages and disadvantages associated with collection and delivery are shown in Box below.

Comparison of Delivery and Collection System.

System	Advantages	Disadvantages
Delivery	• If proper delivery routes, order intervals, and delivery schedules are in place, the total cost of transport will be less. • Deliveries of supplies can be combined with other important scheduled and compulsory visits to the field. Also offers an opportunity to supervise field work. • Drug selection, assembly and packing operations can be scheduled and accomplished efficiently.	• Needs reliable transport facilities. Outright purchase or leasing of vehicles gives rise to high capital and operating costs. • If the delivery route is long, there is the possibility of breakage and loss of quality. • Security lapses may occur due to lack of a responsible officer accompanying goods in many instances. • Health facilities may be closed when the delivery truck arrives, or there may not be a responsible officer on hand to receive. • The delivery truck may be in a hurry to get to the next destination, making it difficult to check for short shipments, damage, and other problems before the truck departs.
Collection	• Provides an opportunity for issuing personnel to meet people from the field and discuss common problems, and for field officers to meet and exchange ideas among themselves. • Frees central-level staff from providing transport facilities to the field. • Provides greater incentive to obtain supplies regularly, since the facility is responsible for collecting supplies. • Allows field personnel to attend to other business in town. • Offers the possibility of a greater choice of methods of transport. • Allows for better checking, handling, and security of goods received.	• Takes up a lot of health facility staff time. • Time may be wasted waiting for assembly of supplies, or supplies might not be ready for collection on the first visit. • Total cost of transport may be high. • Health center personnel may tend to increase the frequency of visits for various reasons.

E. TRANSPORT

1. Transport is frequently the least reliable link in the distribution system and is often a source of great frustration. Transport mangers are responsible for ensuring that drugs are not damaged during transit and ensuring safe and timely delivery.

2. Transport planning requires the selection of appropriate means of transport and the procurement and maintenance of vehicles or other conveyances. Issues to be considered include:

   i. Using private sector alternative

   ii. Planning transport system improvements

   iii. Acquiring and disposing of vehicles

   iv. Managing vehicle use

   v. Maintaining vehicles

   vi. Maintaining drug quality during transport

3. Transport managers should make the best use of available transport through careful route planning and delivery scheduling, and they need to carefully consider private-sector alternatives.

4. Where third-party carriers are used, distributors should develop written agreements with carriers to ensure that appropriate measures are taken to safeguard pharmaceutical products, including maintaining appropriate documentation and records.

F. DELIVERY SCHEDULES

Good planning is needed to ensure that each facility receives supplies regularly and on time. For example, an intermediate store may be responsible for forty clinical facilities with a delivery interval of one month. The total time required to supply all these facilities must not exceed one month. If analysis shows that a longer period is required to supply all facilities, then the delivery schedule must be changed or additional transport resources acquired.

When determining the appropriate delivery intervals for each store and health facility, consider the following factors:

1. Storage Capacity of Primary, Intermediate, and Health Facility Stores: Deliveries must never exceed the holding capacity of any store. This is more likely to occur with irregular or infrequent deliveries.

2. Increased Transport Costs per Unit Supplied for Deliveries to Small, Remote Facilities: An obvious solution is to supply these areas infrequently. The disadvantage is that their policy increases maximum stock levels at these facilities and may also increase the risk of stock outs.

3. Efficient Vehicle Usage: If delivery intervals are too frequent vehicles may travel half empty. If delivery intervals are long, large vehicles will be needed. Vehicles owned by the health service may stand idle for much of the time.

4. Climatic Factors: It may be impossible to deliver to some faculties at certain times of the year, Delivery frequency and volume must be scheduled to work around interruptions caused by rainy seasons or other recurring climatic constraints.

G. COMMUNICATION

1. Good communications are essential to a drug distribution system. Where reliable telecommunications networks and postal services do not exist, especially in rural areas, staff

often has to travel long distances to deliver or collect reports and requisitions. These journeys should be combined with supervisory activities, but often they are not.

2. Good telecommunications reduce the need for travel, save staff time, and reduce wear and tear on vehicles. Maximum use should be made of the telecommunications resources available, and by making appropriate investments in communications technology such as mobile phones, internet, GPS.

3. Where feasible, consideration should be given to adding technology, such as global positioning system (GPS), electronic tracking devices and engine-kill buttons to vehicles, which would enhance the security of pharmaceutical products while in the vehicle.

IV. DISTRIBUTION OF PHARMACEUTICALS/SUPPLY CHAIN IN THE HOSPITAL

The Central Supply Department (CSD)/medical store of the hospital is that unit which provides professional supplies and equipment to all specialized departments. The departments commonly served include out-patient departments or clinics, wards and the operation theatres. Store-in-charge is responsible to manage the department.

A. FUNCTIONS OF THE STORE-IN-CHARGE/PHARMACIST

1. Purchasing, receiving, storing of supplies.

2. Dispensing and distributing supplies to various sections.

3. Inventory and accounting for all supplies received and distributed.

4. Quality assurance of products.

5. Interacting with various professionals involved in health care to cater to their specific needs and for better operational efficiency.

6. For each ward agreement should be reached with nurses and clinicians for those items, which are to be held as stock. Stock levels should be determined from analysis of previous issues and agreed with nursing staff.

7. A ward stock list should be prepared.

B. DISTRIBUTION OF PHARMACEUTICALS TO WARDS/FLOORS

1. A copy of the ward stock list should be made available to nursing staff who will be responsible for obtaining stock supplies, and to prescribers servicing the ward.

2. Written guidelines should be provided on how stock supplies of medicines are to be obtained from the pharmacy together with nurses' responsibilities for signing approved requisition documents i.e.:

   i. An order in writing on approved documents (indent) signed by a registered nurse; or other professionally qualified person in-charge of ward.

   ii. In accordance with a standing order signed by such a person, requiring the stock of medicines to be maintained at a stated level by regular planned replenishment.

   iii. Separate procedures should be provided for Schedule X drugs. For details see section on Handling of Schedule X Drugs.

   iv. When stock is issued without a written order in an emergency, the written order should be furnished within 24 hours of the issue of the product, and

   v. The out-patient pharmacy obtains the medicines from the Hospital Pharmacy against an indent. The supplies from the pharmacy may be as bulk supply.

3. Procedures should define normal action to be taken by pharmaceutical staff for routine stock replacement and action to be taken in the case of incomplete documentation or other queries. Any item temporarily out-of-stock should be supplied as soon as possible.

4. A record must be kept for a minimum stipulated period of 2 years of the quantity supplied of each item and the requisition must be dated and signed.

5. Procedures should be agreed upon for the return of empty stock packs to deter potential misuses such as empty MDI canister, cartridges, empty vial of antirabies vaccine.

6. Procedures should be established to ensure that adequate control of issues is maintained and that regular review of stock ranges are carried out to minimize wastage and overstocking.

7. Regular stock checking by pharmacy personnel should be undertaken at least two-monthly to ensure that stock rotation is maintained in all the hospital medicine storage areas.

8. Procedures should be agreed with nursing staff to allow pharmacist's/or his assistant access to medicine storage facilities with the prior agreement of the nurse-in-charge or other responsible person.

9. Procedures should ensure that a thorough stock-check is carried out prior to topping-up to agreed stock levels.

10. After the drawing up of the topping-up list by pharmacist's, the signature of the nurse-in-charge or other responsible person should be sought either before returning to the pharmacy or on receipt of the stock medicines on a computer printed requisition/packing note.

11. Stock should not be returned to the pharmacy without the agreement of the nurse-in-charge or other responsible person. A written record of its removal should be made on the topping-up list.

C. TRANSPORT AND DELIVERIES TO OTHER HEALTH FACILITIES

1. Pharmacists should ensure that transport is speedy and conditions are sufficient to maintain medicine quality. In particular, cold-chain procedures should be documented and strictly enforced.

2. Products must only be dispatched on valid issue voucher. The receipt of delivery order and the dispatch of goods must be documented (Appendix 6).

3. Supplies and records must include a document stating
   i. The date, the name(s) of the sub-health facility and address
   ii. The product description e.g., name, dosage form and strength, batch number, expiry date and quantity
   iii. The name and address of the supplier and addressee
   iv. The transport and storage conditions

4. Suitable packaging materials must be used to protect the integrity of products dispatched and should be indelibly and clearly labeled.

5. Dispatch procedures should be established and documented taking into account the nature of the materials and pharmaceutical products concerned and any special storage precautions that might be required.

6. Medicine and scheduled products should be transported safely (see below):

7. If third party distributors are utilized, the pharmacist must ensure that the third party distributor is informed of standard operating procedures and trained to handle delivery

of pharmaceutical products and the suitability of the third party distributor to handle pharmaceutical products and ensure adherence to the procedures.

8. All records should be readily accessible and available on request.

D. TRANSPORTING DRUGS SAFELY

Aim is to ensure safe and timely delivery and prevent accidents.

1. It is essential that adequate precautions are taken against spillage, breakage or theft. The drugs are properly packed. Empty spaces in partly filled cartons or crates should be filled with newspaper, straw, wood shavings or loose material to stop contents from rattling about and prevent cartons from being crushed.

2. Their identification is not lost.

3. They do not contaminate, and are not contaminated by, other products or materials.

4. They are secure and not subjected to unacceptable degrees of heat, cold, light, rain, moisture or other adverse influence, nor to attack by micro-organisms or pests.

5. The cold chain, if necessary, is preserved. Thermo labile products must be stored and dispatched under suitable conditions and in suitable containers to preserve the integrity of the product and maintain the cold chain.

6. Special care should be exercised when using dry ice in cold chain. In addition, to observing special precautions, it must be ensured that the material or product does not come in to the contact with dry ice, as this may adversely affect the product quality by freezing.

7. Where appropriate temperature monitoring devices to monitor temperature during transportation should be used and records should be available.

8. Load vehicles carefully and systematically first-out/last-in to save time when unloading and prevent damage.

9. Secure vehicle doors to prevent losses or theft and stay near the vehicle to guard against theft.

10. Start early in the day and drive with care, especially on hazardous roads and avoid nighttime driving.

8 | Quantification of Medical Supplies

Drugs and medical supplies are dispensed at the cutting edge level of the interface between the public health system and the people. Availability or lack of availability brings either credit or discredit to the public health system. The availability and accessibility of medicines/especially at public health facilities thus become a determinant of the quality of health care and in private systems means loss of revenue. To ensure constant availability of drugs and medical supplies, it is of the utmost importance that store management at health facilities are organized efficiently.

I. QUANTIFICATION OF MEDICINES NEEDS

Drug needs can be quantified by using one or a combination of four standard methods. Quantification involves estimating the quantities of specific drugs needed for procurement. The quantification methods described in this chapter are normally used to forecast needs for an annual or semiannual procurement. The goal is to maintain the most cost-effective balance between service levels and inventory costs. The most precise method for forecasting drug usage is the consumption based approach, provided the source data are complete, accurate and properly adjusted for stock out periods and anticipated changes in demand and use.

This section indicates the broad steps and various processes involved in estimation of drug needs but these processes are to be understood in the overall background of the rationale of proper inventory management in the overall scheme of management of drug supply.

Quantification is defined as, the process "to determine the quantity" or "to express a property that is measurable". Quantification of medical supplies involves estimating how much of specific item is needed and the financial means are required.

Health Facility (HF)/Districts are required to estimate their own supply needs within a given budget as part of the decentralization of planning and budgeting activities. The shift from a push (where supply needs are determined centrally) to a pull system (where supply needs are determined locally) requires HF/districts to determine the quantities of essential supplies required to deliver the essential services within their budget allocation.

Very often the need will be greater than the allocated budget, it is, therefore, necessary to rationally adjust the quantification to within the allocated budget. This manual describes the process for quantifying and reconciling needs to the budget.

II. WHY QUANTIFY?

1. To avoid stock-outs and ensure continuous availability of essential supplies.
2. To avoid wastage due to overstocking.

3. To make the best use of scarce resources and to budget within your means to facilitate central bulk purchasing by providing sufficiently detailed information from health facilities to allow central orders to be placed well in advance.

III. ACTION PLANNING

Quantification of medical supplies is part of the planning process for the annual action plans. This should be integrated with contraceptives, drugs, laboratory supplies, vaccines and other medical supply items being quantified by a working group of all concerned parties following the methods described in this manual.

The working group should be chaired by the Chief Medical Officer (CMO) or Medical Superintendent/ Head. The group should include, at least, staff with expertise in drugs, laboratory, vaccines and family planning, either from the districts office, from the hospital or a health centre. The most experienced and qualified person in each field should be used.

The following is required for the action plan:

1. That the most essential items required to deliver the appropriate package of care are included.

2. That each item is quantified based on reliable data.

3. That the quantities have been adjusted for stock on hand and wastage.

4. Programmatic and emphasis changes have been considered.

5. That items and quantities have been prioritized keeping in mind demand behaviour (see below) and adjusted to the budget allocation.

6. That estimates have been validated.

7. That the quantification form has been completed.

Illustration of Broad Concepts of Quantification

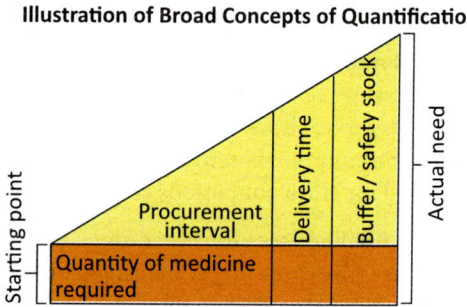

Demand behaviour—Trends of Medicine consumption

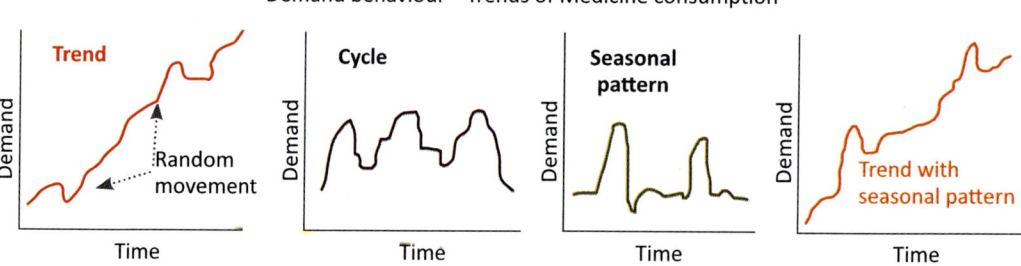

IV. THE QUANTIFICATION PROCESS

A. PREPARATORY PHASE

Step 1: Name the person responsible for coordinating the process

The quantification process needs someone to be specifically responsible with authority to carry through all the required activities, and must understand the methodologies used. The suggested person is the Manager Planning.

Step 2: Form the working group

This should include pharmacy, lab, public health nurse, manager planning and others as thought necessary by the HF/district.

Step 3: Agree on specific objectives of the working group

The ultimate objective of quantifying medical supplies is to ensure that appropriate supplies are available for the expected case load of patients and to promote the rational use of these supplies. More specific and smaller objectives however need to be set in order to achieve this.

Step 4: Choose quantification method for each group of medical supply items based on the most accurate data source available

There is no single best way to quantify medical supply requirements. The methods described in this manual are thought to be the simplest and most appropriate to the current situation in the State.

Step 5: Prepare an action plan: list the tasks, estimate cost for exercise, estimate time requirements

Step 6: Allocate tasks amongst the members of the working group

It is important to ensure that everyone understands what is expected of them and the time scale within which the exercise must be completed. The person leading the working group should co-ordinate and keep in touch with the working group.

B. QUANTIFICATION PHASE

Using the Drugs and Therapeutics Committee:

Step 7: List health problems to be treated, tested for and prevented at health facilities in the Health facility (HF)/district

Deciding which health problems are to be catered for at each level of care is a matter of health policy and must be decided taking into account national guidelines. The drugs and therapeutics should co-ordinate with the working group to come up with such a list.

Step 8: Select appropriate items required for each health problem to draw up an essential medical supplies list for the Health facility (HF)/District

Drawing up a list of "essential items" is an important step in maximizing the impact of the limited funds that are available to ensure that the maximum number of patients are diagnosed, treated or serviced.

It is important not to forget important items such as syringes, needles and water for injection. Guidelines on selection on essential medical supplies are given in Chapter on Pharmaceutical Supply Management.

Step 9: Collect data on all of the items, quantify, cost and reconcile to budget

The details of this process are described in sections VI and VII. Reconciliation of needs and the budget allocation by a systematic method will allow rational decisions to be made with a minimum impact on health care provision.

Step 10: Feedback results to Quantification Team and Health Management Team

The quantification will only be effective if results are fed back to the quantification team and the management.

Step 11: Evaluate how the quantification process went

The ultimate objectives of quantifying medical supplies are to ensure that appropriate supplies are available for the expected case load of patients and to promote the rational use of these supplies. However, the extent to which these objectives are achieved cannot be used to evaluate the effectiveness of quantification, as quantification is only one component of the medical supply management system. Selection, financing, procurement, distribution, storage and use at all levels also have to be carried out effectively in order to achieve the ultimate objectives.

Step 12: Inform medical personnel on quantification reconciliation decisions

The quantification process has been based on certain assumptions and reconciliation will have involved making some choices. It is important that the medical personnel are informed of these decisions, so as to be able to reflect them in their practice.

Step 13: Provide training in stores procedures and rational use of drugs and other supplies

After quantifying the medical supply item needs, it is likely that they will be greater than the budget. Improving the stores management to reduce wastage and improving the rational use of supplies, will ensure that the maximum number of patients will receive the items that they require.

Irrational use of supplies and poor stores management will deprive patients of the items they need in their treatment.

V. QUANTIFICATION METHODS

Drug needs can be quantified by using one or a combination of four standard methods. Quantification involves estimating the quantities of specific medical supplies needed for procurement. Most quantification exercises also estimate the financial requirements to purchase the medical supplies.

1. **Consumption method**

   The consumption method uses records of past consumption of individual items (adjusted for stock-outs, losses and growth) to project future need.

2. **Morbidity method**

   Morbidity looks at the frequency of illness. The morbidity method estimates the need for specific items based on the expected number of attendances, the incidence of common diseases, and standard treatment guidelines for the diseases considered.

3. **Adjusted consumption method**

   The adjusted consumption method uses data on disease incidence, consumption or utilization, and/or expenditures from a standard supply system and extrapolates the consumption or utilization rates to the target supply system, based on population coverage or service level to be provided. The area from which the data is taken from must have a good supply system and be comparable in terms of morbidity, types of facility and prescribing habits.

4. **Service-level projection of budget requirements**

   Service-level projection of budget requirements uses the average medical supply procurement cost per attendance or bed-day in different types of health facilities in a standard system to project drug cost in similar types of facilities in the target system. This method does not estimate quantities of individual items.

Two main methods for quantification, consumption and morbidity are described as under.

VI. DETAILS OF CONSUMPTION METHOD

The general method for drugs, family planning and laboratory are very similar and are calculated by the following calculation steps:

1. Total consumption over a period
2. Number of days out-of-stock
3. Number of months in stock/test available
4. Adjusted average monthly consumption
5. Lead time
6. Safety stock
7. Suggested quantity to order
8. Total upward adjustment for growth and losses
9. Stock on hand + stock on order (but not yet received)
10. Number of months stock on hand + stock on order
11. Order quantity
12. Price
13. Value of proposed order
14. % cost (ABC analysis)
15. Adjusted order quantity
16. Adjusted value

Step 1. Selection of Essential Medical Supplies

Essential medical supplies should be selected by the local Drugs and Therapeutics Committee (DTC), and should be reviewed at least once a year.

For drugs, the Essential Medicines List (EML) and Standard Treatment Guidelines (STGs) can be used as a starting point for selection of essential medical supplies.

Factors that should be considered in drug selection are:

1. Decide which conditions you are going to treat.
2. Selection should be based on scientific proof of effectiveness and safety.
3. Select the minimum number of drugs needed to treat prevalent diseases. Avoid unnecessary duplication and close similarities in drugs or dosage forms.
4. Compare newly released products with products with known efficacy and safety, include only if found to have distinct advantages over products currently in use.
5. Include combination products only when they provide true benefit over individual use of each component.
6. When several alternatives are available, select drugs with clear "drug of choice" indications for the prevalent diseases in the country setting.

7. When several alternatives are available, also consider which is the least expensive.

8. Evaluate the administrative cost impact of products in terms of ease of purchase, storage, distribution, dosage units needed, etc.

9. Select drug for which adequate standards of quality have been established.

10. Contraindications, precautions and adverse effect should be thoroughly investigated and evaluated in order to obtain benefit/risk ratio for the product.

11. Drugs should be referred by the generic name only when published in the formulary.

12. Level of use – it should be considered what level of prescriber can prescribe each drug. Proper prescribing is dependent on proper diagnosis. The level of training of a prescriber limits the types of conditions that can be treated by that person and hence the drug prescribed.

13. The storage requirements and the unit size that the supply is available in should also be considered. For details see chapter on Pharmaceutical Supply Management.

Step 2. Total Consumption in a Period

The total consumption in a period informs how much has been used in a specific period. When quantifying, it is best to use the period of 1 year so as to eliminate any seasonal variation.

Step 3. Number of Days out-of-Stock

This is calculated by adding up the number of days that the item was out-of-stock, i.e. the stock level is nil or zero, from the stock control card.

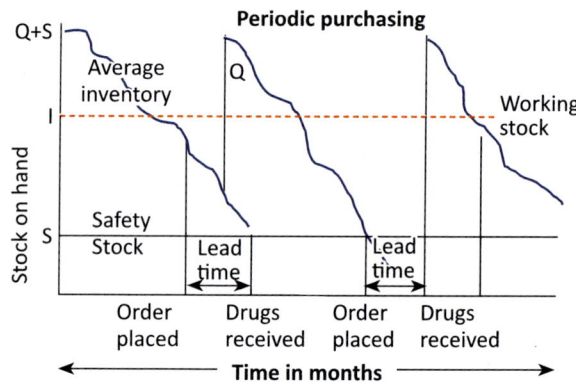

Step 4. Average Monthly Consumption

The average monthly consumption is a measure of how much of a supply item is used in an average month. The adjusted monthly consumption is similar, but an adjustment is made to account for any time that the item was unavailable.

Step 5. Filling the Supply Pipeline

The supply pipeline refers to stock levels within the supply system and the number of supply points at each level that are required to be filled.

The number of levels, the frequency of requisition and delivery, and the amount of safety stock at each level all influence the amount that is needed to fill the pipeline and, hence the amount that must be procured when a programme is started or expanded. Underestimation of stock in the pipeline is a common cause of programme failure, particularly when a revolving medical supply fund has been planned.

Step 6. Lead Time

When you decide that you need some medical supplies, they will not arrive for some time; you need to take this into account. This is the lead time, and starts from when the decision to order drugs is started until the time the drugs are available to the patient. e.g., if it takes 2 months for your orders to arrive, the lead time is 2 months. The lead time should be stated as a number of months of stock and should be as realistic as possible. If it is variable (may vary from 15 days to months) consider the longest time as lead time or take average time as lead time.

Step 7. Safety Stock

Safety stock is an amount of stock that is kept in reserve to allow for an item to be unavailable from the supplier and also to account for sudden increases in demand.

The minimum safety stock needed to avoid a stock-out is the quantity of stock used, on average, during the lead time e.g., if it takes 2 months to get supplied, it is the amount of stock that would be used during a 2 month period.

It is calculated by multiplying the lead time (LT) by the adjusted average monthly consumption (C_A). i.e. in the example above the average monthly consumption $C_A \times 2$.

$$SS = C_A \times LT$$

If the lead time is set high, the safety stock and the overall stock levels will rise, therefore, it may not be financially feasible to have very large safety stocks. For details see inventory management, service level and safety stock requirements.

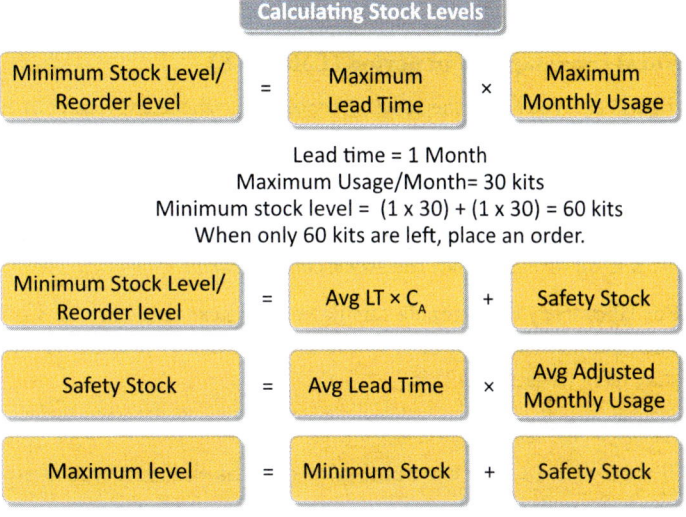

Calculating Stock Levels

| Minimum Stock Level/ Reorder level | = | Maximum Lead Time | × | Maximum Monthly Usage |

Lead time = 1 Month
Maximum Usage/Month= 30 kits
Minimum stock level = (1 x 30) + (1 x 30) = 60 kits
When only 60 kits are left, place an order.

| Minimum Stock Level/ Reorder level | = | Avg LT × C_A | + | Safety Stock |

| Safety Stock | = | Avg Lead Time | × | Avg Adjusted Monthly Usage |

| Maximum level | = | Minimum Stock | + | Safety Stock |

Avg - Average

Step 8. Adjusting for Losses and Programme Growth

Inevitably, some items will be lost due to damage, spoilage, expiration, and theft. If such losses are not considered in quantification and procurement, stock-outs are likely to result. To prevent shortages, a percentage can be added to allow for losses when quantifying requirements. Not everything is equally at risk for loss – for example some are more attractive to thieves than others. If it is possible to identify them, it may be feasible to adjust the quantities for those items by a higher percentage rather than applying the same adjustment to all items. One strategy is to allow a loss percentage only for vital items, accepting the risk of stock-outs for other items. Clearly, it is in the best interests of the health system to make every effort to control loss and wastage.

In a supply system in which patient utilization or the number of facilities is growing, it is reasonable to assume that the drug consumption will increase. In such situations, estimated quantities can be increased by a percentage corresponding to the rate of growth.

Step 9. Number of Months Stock on Hand

The number of months of stock in hand gives you an indication of whether an item is overstocked or not. If the number of months of stock on hand is greater than 3 months stock for district stores or greater than 2 months stock for a health facility, than the item is overstocked.

If the number of months of stock is greater than 6 months, then something needs to be done to reduce the stock holding, such as arranging for the item to be transferred.

The number of months of stock on hand is calculated by dividing the months of stock on hand by the average monthly consumption.

$$\text{Period of stock on hand} = \frac{\text{months of stock on hand}}{\text{average monthly consumption}}$$

VII. QUANTIFICATION OF DRUGS CALCULATION SHEET

Using the consumption based quantification calculation sheet (see Annexure I):

Columns B, C and D should be filled in for all the items which have been selected for the HF/district.

Total consumption in period (Column E)

This is derived from the stock control card, where they exist or from annual test statistics for labs where no stock control cards are kept

Number of days out-of-stock (Column F)

This is calculated by adding up the number of days that the item was out-of-stock, i.e. the stock level is nil or zero, from the stock control card.

For laboratory consumable calculations, where there are no stock control cards, it is preferable to use column G instead of F, where the number of months the test was available is recorded. You may have to estimate this.

Number of months in stock/test available (Column G)

This column records the number of months the item was in stock or the number of months the test was available.

The number of months in stock is calculated from column F. The number of days needs to be converted into the number of months.

$$\text{\# Months the item was out-of-stock} = \frac{\text{column F}}{30.5}$$

$$\text{\# Months in stock} = \frac{12 - \text{column F}}{30.5}$$

(30.5 is the average number of days in 1 month)

For the laboratory, the number of months the test was available is taken from the monthly reports or log books and entered directly.

Adjusted average monthly consumption (Column H)

The adjusted monthly consumption is the consumption per month with an upward adjustment being made for the time when the item was unavailable for use. For example, if the item was only available for 10 months, the average monthly consumption should be divided by 10 and NOT 12.

An adjustment is made for what would have been used of that item if it had been available for the whole year.

This is calculated by dividing the total consumption for 1 year by the number of months the item was in stock.

$$\text{Adjusted average monthly consumption} = \frac{\text{total consumption in period}}{\text{of months in stock/test available}} = \frac{\text{column E}}{\text{column G}}$$

Lead time (column I)

An estimate needs to be made for the average time it takes to receive your supplies. The lead time may be different for different items. If it is known that particular item is difficult to get and is often not available, it has a longer lead time.

Safety stock (Column J)

The safety stock is the amount of stock you want to keep in reserve for unexpected increases in demand and to have an allowance for delays in receiving the next supplies. This is the level of stock below which the stock levels should not fall. It is used to try to avoid stock-outs.

It is important to consider the increased cost of a large safety stock. The safety stock should therefore reflect true uncertainties in lead time or monthly consumption. A larger safety stock is needed for fast moving stable items. You should not keep a large safety stock of slow movers or supplies with a short expiry date (e.g. antisera and chemistry kits).

Safety stock can be calculated using the following formula:

Safety Stock = Average Monthly Consumption × Lead Time

If your average monthly consumption is 50 containers of aspirin and the lead time is 2 months, then the safety stock would be 50 × 2 = 100 containers of aspirin.

Suggested quantity to order (Column K)

This is the sum of the amount of medical supplies required for the procurement period and the safety stock. Before finalizing the suggested order quantity, the stock on hand and the stock on order should be considered. If an item is highly overstocked, then the suggested order quantity should be reduced.

If the procurement period is 12 months then:

Suggested Order Quantity = 12 × C_A + SS

C_A- Average monthly consumption

SS- Safety stock

Total upward adjustment (column L)

1. *Adjustment for Expected Changes in Consumption Patterns*

   If there is an expected change in usage patterns e.g. if the number of TB cases is on the increase then the percentage increase should be estimated and the amounts increased accordingly

   For family planning, an adjustment needs to be made for an increase in the number of clients that are expected for the next year.

2. *Adjust for Losses and Wastage*

   There will be a certain percentage of wastage due to pilferage, expiration, damages, spillages, however, this should be kept to a minimum, if supplies are managed correctly. A higher figure should be estimated for slow moving items with short expiry dates.

   Add the percentages for programmatic change, losses and adjustments and enter in column L.

Calculate the required adjustment by multiplying the % increased by the adjusted annual requirement

> Total upward adjustment = Expected changes in pattern + Losses & wastage

Example:

i. **Changes in consumption** – are there any expected changes in consumption expected, an increase or a decrease?

    Make an estimation of any programme growth (shrinkage, which would be a negative figure):

    In this example it was estimated that there would be a growth of 5%

    % Adjustment for programme growth: 5%

ii. **Adjust for losses** (breakage's expiry of stock, theft, wastage of medicines or laboratory reagents (this may vary for different reagents, e.g. volatile substances will have a high wastage), irrational use. The adjustment for losses should be less than 10%. Fill in the table below to estimate your losses:

	%
Breakages:	2
Expiry:	1
Theft:	1
Waste/spillage:	1
Irrational use:	1
Other losses:	0.5
Total loses:	6.5

Make an estimation of the total upward adjustment necessary by adding the 2 adjustments.

Total upward adjustment: 5+6.5 = 11.5%   (= column L)

The same adjustment might be made for all products or adjustments might be different for different products.

Adjusted order quantity (Column M)

The expected annual requirement is adjusted for changes in consumption patterns and wastage and losses. This includes losses due to pilferage, expiration, damages, spillage's, etc.

$$\text{Adjusted order quantity} = \text{suggested order quantity} \times \frac{100 + \% \text{ adjustment}}{100}$$

$$= \text{Column J} \times \frac{100 + \text{column L}}{100}$$

Stock on hand + stock on order (but not yet received) (column N)

This is the stock which you have in stock now plus the stock which has been ordered, but has not yet arrived (be careful to include all items that you know that will be made available to you)

This need to be considered when making the order quantity, as above, and the suggested order quantity might be needed to be reduced. It should be considered when you look at the order quantity – there might be sufficient stock already for next year!

In which case the suggested order quantity should be reduced.

Number of months stock on hand or ordered (column O)

This is estimated by dividing the stock on hand or ordered by the average monthly consumption

i.e. Number of months stock on hand/ordered $= \dfrac{\text{Stock on hand/ordered}}{\text{Adjusted average monthly consumption}}$

$$= \dfrac{\text{Column N}}{\text{Column H}}$$

Order quantity (Column P)

If the number of months stock on hand/ordered is large and will last into the next year for which the quantification is being done, then the quantity required should be reduced to take account of this.

For example, if it is October now and it is calculated for quinine injection that there is 7 months stock on hand, then it is not necessary to quantify for 12 months, less is required.

The stock will last for October, November, December, January, February, March, April.

Therefore it is only necessary to quantify for May-December: 8 months plus the safety stock.

An alternative method to adjust the order quantity is to subtract the stock on hand from the adjusted order quantity. The difference will give an approximate order quantity.

It however does not take into account the months between when the quantification is done and the period of the quantification.

If the answer for this subtraction is negative, then you are overstocked and none of this item may be required.

Order quantity is approximately = adjusted order quantity – (stock on hand)

= Column M – Column N

Price (Column Q)

This column contains the price of the item.

If the price of an item is not on the list, then another reputable source of price should be used. Examples are previous invoices, price lists and local price lists.

Care should be taken to check that the price used corresponds to the pack size used in quantification. If there is a discrepancy, an adjustment should be made.

Price should be in Rupees, for ease of calculation.

Value of proposed order (Column R)

The value of the proposed order is the order quantity multiplied by the price for the pack size.

Value of proposed order = order quantity × price for 1 unit

Example glucostix:

Estimating cost of the quantities required = ₹ 30.4 × 17 = ₹ 517

Total value of all items

The total value of all of the requirements should be made by adding up for each item the value of the proposed order for each item, (adding up all **column R's**)

(Column A, S, T and U) is described in section on reconciliation of needs to the budget using ABC and VED analysis.

VIII. MORBIDITY METHOD

For example TB drugs are quantified using an estimate of requirements which is made by looking at the number of patients diagnosed in the previous quarter.

The method should be adapted to make 12 month estimation for the quantification period and then the total requirement for each **drug added into** column P of the quantification table, columns Q-U should be followed in the same way as described using ABC and VED analysis.

Quantification Calculations are Complete!!

Next step is Reconciliation of the Needs to the Budget for Drugs

IX. RECONCILIATION OF NEEDS AND BUDGET

Under ideal conditions, the budget would be adequate to meet the needs estimated. In practice, this is usually not the case. In the first instance the Health facility (HF)/district should argue for the budget required to support your requirements provided your data is reliable and the quantification can be justified. The better is your data, the easier it will be to support your case.

In the event that additional funds are not available or sufficient to meet your needs, the quantities must be reviewed to bring the total order within the ceilings allocated.

Difficult decisions must often be made to reduce the number of medical supply items and/or the quantities of the items until the estimated quantities and costs correspond with the available budget. These reductions may require policy decisions regarding priority diseases, priority age groups, priority facilities for supply, selection of less expensive therapeutic alternatives, and changes to Standard Treatment Guidelines.

This section discusses several approaches to making reductions rationally, using specific tools such as VED (vital, essential, desirable) categories, and ABC analysis details given below. For more details see section on inventory management tools. Another way to provide a foundation for reduction is to cross-check the quantification with another method to find out where the quantified estimate is much higher than necessary based on known morbidity and attendance data or much higher than that in a comparable health system.

X. SELECTIVE INVENTORY CONTROL TOOLS

The importance of a material can be due to its: Cost, Criticality, Availability or Consumption. Drugs are divided according to their health impact into Vital, Essential & Desirable (VED) or by value of consumption or value of items in store, etc. ABC and VED analysis are two commonly used tools for selective inventory control. For details see section on Inventory Management.

Selective inventory control	VED Analysis (Criticality)	ABC Analysis (Cost)

• The importance of a material can be due to its:
 	
  • Cost
  • Criticality
  • Availability
  • Consumption
 	
How do we identify the vital few?
	• V: vital drugs potentially life saving, making supply mandatory, critical to basic health needs.
	
	• E: essential drugs effective against less severe but significant form of illness
	
	• D: desirable drugs used either for minor or self limited disease, BUT least important items.
		A: Supplies accounting for a high percentage of the cost. This includes 10-20% of items which account for 75-80% of expenditure.
		
		B: Supplies accounting for a medium percentage of the cost. This includes 10-20% of items and 10-15% of expenditure.
		
		C: Supplies accounting for a low percentage of the cost. This includes 60-80% of items but only 5-10% of expenditure.

A. VED ANALYSIS

One way to maximize the effectiveness of the health system when funds are limited is to set priorities according to the potential health impact of individual medical supplies. A method of doing this is the VED system, in which all of the items are placed into one of the following three categories:

VITAL items: are potentially life-saving, which have significant withdrawal-side-effects; a health care system needs these supplies in order to function.

ESSENTIAL items: are effective against, or required for the diagnosis of less severe, but nevertheless significant forms of illness, where an alternative might already exist as a vital item: without these supplies the health care system can still function.

DESIRABLE items for minor or self limited illnesses, items which are of questionable efficacy, low priority items with a high cost for a marginal therapeutic or diagnostic advantage.

The steps below summarize some guidelines in applying the VED system. When applying the VED system, not all of the guidelines have to apply to a particular drug in order for it to be categorized as V, E or D.

STEPS OF VED ANALYSIS

1. Each DTC member should classify all the medicines as V,E, or D

2. The results of each member's classification should be compiled and an overall classification agreed in the DTC. VED categories can be written in column A or the quantification calculation sheet. (Annexure I). The DTC should then:

3. Reconsider the proposed order quantities to make sure they are justified.

4. Identify and limit therapeutic duplication

5. Adjust to your budgets or seek more funding using the evidence of needs that you have produced.

6. Examine all the D items and where possible decrease the quantities purchased or eliminate them and reassess the total compared to the budget

7. If necessary reduce quantities, remove and eliminate more items

8. Reduce quantities further:

    "Equal misery system": reduce all quantities by the same percentage until you reach the desired cost reduction.

    "Preferential weighting": protect certain categories (V items), facilities or programmes, reducing some more than others.

9. Reconsider proposed purchase quantities, buying V and E items before D items and ensuring that safety stocks are higher for V and E items

10. Monitor drug ordering and stock levels for V and E items more closely than for D items.

Sample guidelines for VED categories

Characteristics of the drug and target condition	Vital	Essential	Desirable
Occurrence of target condition % of population affected Average number of patients treated per day in an average facility	>5% >5	1-5% 1-5	<1% <1
Severity of target condition Life-threatening Disabling	Yes Yes	Occasionally Occasionally	Rarely Rarely
Therapeutic effect of drug Prevents serious disease Cures serious disease Treats minor, self-limited symptoms and conditions Has proven efficacy Does not have proven efficacy	Yes Yes No Always Never	No Yes Possibly Usually Rarely	No No Yes May be May be

B. ABC ANALYSIS

ABC analysis directs the attention to the few items that account for the majority of the expenditure. This is where there is potential for the greatest saving. An ABC analysis can be performed on items you plan to purchase or items already purchased or consumed.

ABC analysis divides drugs into categories depending on their relative cost. Supplies are classified as:

A: Supplies accounting for a high percentage of the cost. This includes 10-20% of items which account for 75-80% of expenditure.

B: Supplies accounting for a medium percentage of the cost. This includes 10-20% of items and 10-15% of expenditure.

C: Supplies accounting for a low percentage of the cost. This includes 60-80% of items but only 5-10% of expenditure.

STEPS OF ABC ANALYSIS

Full method

Using the ABC analysis forms (Step 1-5 and 6-8) in Annexure II:

Step 1: List all items you have quantified

Step 2: Enter the unit cost

Step 3: Enter consumption/order quantities

Step 4: For each item, calculate the value of the proposed order

Step 5: Calculate the percentage of the total represented by each item.

already performed during quantification methods (Annexure I).

Step 6: Rearrange and rank the items in descending order.

Step 7: Calculate the cumulative percentage

Step 8: Choose cut-offs for the boundaries of A, B, and C.

> A: 10-20% items representing 75-80% of the funds
>
> B: 10-20% items representing 15-20% of the funds
>
> C: 60-80% of the items representing 5-10% of funds

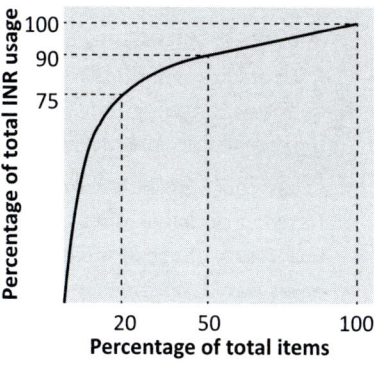

Step 9: (optional): Present the results graphically with cumulative percentages on the vertical y-axis and the drugs listed in descending rank on the x-axis.

Step 10: Desirable (D) should not appear in class A, i.e. a large proportion of funds should not be spent on non-essential items. Vital (V) and essential items (E) can appear in either A, B or C, it is not important that a small amount of money is spent on a vital item.

Step 11: The following are some of the questions you could ask about class A drugs, and make decisions over reducing use and hence requirements, thus allowing budgetary savings:

– Is there a lower cost alternative?

– Is there inappropriate prescribing or use of this item, that could be improved?

– Can a smaller quantity of this item be given to the patient?

Step 12: The results may be presented graphically by plotting the percentage of total cumulative value on the vertical or y axis and the number of items (accounting for this cumulative value) on the horizontal or x axis.

SHORT METHOD

Step 1: Using the calculation sheet for recording consumption data, add up the total value of all items.

Step 2: Calculate the % spent on each of the items and enter this in **column S** of the quantification calculation sheet.

$$\% \text{ cost (of each item)} = \frac{\text{value of proposed order for that item}}{\text{total value of all proposed quantities and items}} \times 100$$

$$= \frac{R}{\text{total value of all items}} \times 100$$

Step 3: Identify the "A" items as those which account for the largest percentages calculated in step 2 and entered in column S. Mark these items as "A" in **column A,** next to the VED category.

Step 4: Consider reducing the quantities of A items:

– which are non-essential (reduce or remove)

– where there is a cheaper alternative available (decrease this item and increase the quantity of the cheaper alternative)

XI. VALIDATION OF ESTIMATES

1. Since there will be some imprecision in the estimates no matter how rigorously the appropriate quantification methods are followed, it is always useful to check the estimates with a different quantification method. The two sets of data can then be compared to see which appears to be more realistic, considering the reliability of source data used for the two estimates.

2. Cross-checking is a fundamental step to reconcile procurement quantities with available funds. It is also useful to cross-check consumption with theoretical need to get an idea of the rationality of use of medical supplies in the system. For example, if the supply system usually bases purchases on past consumption, cross-checking for high-volume, high-cost drugs using another method may reveal targets for interventions to promote more rational use.

3. Once the quantification is complete by the consumption method, it is important to validate whether the estimates are realistic.

4. Choose class A items for the ABC analysis to validate your estimations. A items are responsible for most of the budget, therefore validating a number of these items will validate a large proportion of the budget. e.g., validate the consumption method for quantifying drugs by making some estimates based on the morbidity method. For example from morbidity data and standard treatments of malaria, make an estimate of your chloroquine requirements and see if this matches with your consumption estimates. Morbidity looks at the frequency of illness. The morbidity method estimates the need for specific items based on the expected number of attendances, the incidence of common diseases, and standard treatment guidelines for the diseases considered. If the number of expected malaria cases in 1 year can be estimated and this multiplied by the number of chloroquine tablets in a standard course (10), then this will give an estimate of the chloroquine requirement based on morbidity.

Reconciliation of Needs & Budget

Use the method of quantification best suited to the available data- morbidity method, if morbidity data are available and Standard Treatment Guidelines (STGs) are followed, or consumption method, if there are no morbidity data and STGs are not followed.

Use VED analysis to identify the most essential medicines, especially if there is insufficient budget to finance all medicines needs.

The DTC should assist the procurement group to do this once each department has submitted the yearly quantification of medicines needs.

Guiding Purchases with the VED system and ABC analysis

- Often requirements exceed available resources. Adjustments may have to be made cautiously if there is not enough budget to procure all the medicines needed.

- Under these constraints, requests need to be revised, but the process for doing so is frequently haphazard. Reduce purchase quantity in proportion to the health impact, rather than in proportion to the quantities requested.

- Consider deleting/reducing 'D' items in A category or reducing/replacing 'E' items for which equally effective cheaper alternative is available.

- The VED system helps to minimize these and other distortions in the procurement process, and thus maximize the health impact of available funds.

Annexure I. Consumption based quantification calculation sheet

VED	ITEM	Form and strength of item	Unit size	Total consumption in period	Days out-of-stock	Months in stock	Adjusted Average Monthly Consumption	Lead time	Safety stock
A	B	C	D	E	F	G	H	I	J
				#pack of unit size (column D)	day	months	#units of pack size (column D)	months	#units of pack size (column D)
						$12 - \dfrac{F}{30.5}$ (or records)	$\dfrac{E}{G}$	Delivery schedule experience	$I \times H$

Annexure I. Consumption based quantification calculation sheet contd...

Suggested Quantity to order	Total upward adjustment	Adjusted order quality	Stock on hand stock ordered (but not yet received)	#months on hand or stock ordered	Order quality	Price (Rs.)	Value of proposed order	% cost (ABC analysis)	Adjusted order qty	Adjusted value
K	L	M	N	O	P	Q	R	S	T	U
#pack of unit size (column D)	%	#pack of unit size (column D)	#pack of unit size (column D)	months	# pack of unit size (column D)	Rs.	Rs.			
$(12 \times H) + J$	see manual	$\dfrac{K \times (100+I)}{100}$	Stock cards/ books	$\dfrac{N}{H}$	considering columns M, N & O [M-N]	price list	$P \times Q$	$\dfrac{R \times 100}{\text{total value of all items}}$		$T \times Q$

Annexure II. ABC analysis Step 1-5

Product description	Form	Unit price in quantification/ tender (₹)	Total units on order	Value (₹)	% Total value

Total value

ABC Value ANALYSIS- Step 6-8 (rearranged in descending % of total value)

Product description	Form	% of total value	Cumulative % of value	A, B, or C

9 | Medical Stores Management

The goals of medical store management are to manage the reliable movement of supplies from source to user in the most expeditious and economical way without loss, damage, theft, or wastage. The primary purpose of a store is to receive, hold and dispatch stock. The integrated process is known as materials management and is implemented through inventory control and warehouse management systems. A warehouse management system monitors the physical flow of goods within the system which includes receipts, storage and issues. Though level of sophistication of medical stores varies widely and each store approaches its system and documentation differently, the basic features and principles presented in this chapter remain the same.

I. RECEIVING AND ARRANGING COMMODITIES

A. RECEIVING HEALTH COMMODITIES

1. Stock must be received in a separate receiving area and examined for damaged containers. The pharmaceutical storage area must be under the control of the pharmacy medical store. Make sure at least two staff members receive and check supplies.

2. Check the delivery note, packing list and contents against a copy of the order.

3. Check and physically verify the contents and number of boxes against the packing list.

4. Check the outer and inner packaging to make sure it is intact and for signs of damage, for example, spots, breakages, leaks, missing labels, tape or lids..

5. Check labels are legible and include complete information, for example, the approved name, strengths, storage instructions, manufacturer's details, expiry date and unique identifiers present or not (article code, Govt. supply stamp, other code, if any).

6. Check that all spare parts, accessories, instruction manuals, and warranty documents are included.

7. On receipt each incoming delivery should be checked against the relevant purchase order and each container should be physically verified e.g., by the label description, batch number, type of pharmaceutical product and quantity. Any discrepancy should be documented (Appendix 2).

8. Report any problems to the supplier and the carrier immediately, explaining the nature of the problem, for example under-supply or damaged goods. (See Appendix 2) Do not use damaged goods.

9. Systematic checking involves following steps:

   i. Compactness of packing: Loosely packed good will produce noise. Check boxes/cartons in such cases.

   ii. Weight: Standard shopper packs would almost weight the same

   iii. Some small cartons may contain less quantity, or may even be empty. Check in case of doubt.

10. Store in-charge should be responsible whether or not personally undertakes the task.

11. All deliveries should be formally received whether during or outside working hours (Appendix 3).

12. All relevant documentation must be recorded (Appendix 3) and all stock must be checked for quantity, quality, type, condition and expiry dates.

13. **Ensure remaining 75% shelf life at the time of receiving or as per policy of the state/ hospital.**

14. There must be a system for the recognition of and the prompt and correct handling by the store in-charge/pharmacist of Schedule X substances and for those products requiring storage at specific temperature ranges. Delivery of Schedule X medicines must be made directly to the medical store/pharmacy.

15. All applicable documentation and receipts for medicines and scheduled substances must be retained for a period of ten years after the date of the last entry made therein. Sample receiving report is shown in Appendix 3.

16. In case a register is kept by computer, a computer printout must be made monthly, dated, signed and filed (Appendix 4).

17. When you receive health commodities
    i. Ensure there is sufficient storage space.
    ii. Prepare and clean the areas used for receiving and storing the products.
    iii. Inspect packages for damaged or expired products.

18. If products are damaged or expired then
    i. Separate the damaged or expired stock from the usable stock.
    ii. If damage or expiry is discovered while the supplier/supplier vendor/delivery truck is still at your site, refuse to accept the products and note the problem(s) on the delivery note.
    iii. If damage or expiry is discovered after the supplier/supplier vendor/delivery truck has departed, follow your facility's procedures for handling damaged or expired stock.

19. If products are not damaged or expired then
    i. Count the number of units for each product received and compare with supply order/ issue voucher.
    ii. Record the date and quantity received on stock card and bin card[14] (Appendix 5).
    iii. Ensure remaining 75% shelf life at the time of receiving or as per policy of the state hospital.
    iv. Ensure the expiry date is visibly marked on every package or unit (e.g. Aug 2019).
        For example may put a conspicuous red star or a similar mark on the labels of all items that have an expiry date within the current year.
    v. Arrange products in the storage area to facilitate the first-to-expire, first-out (FEFO) procedure (See section on stock rotation).

Bin Card

Product Name _____   Pack Size: _____

Balance Brought Forward: _____   Date: _____

Date	In	Out	Total on Hand

---

14 Bin card: Card that records receipts, issues, and balances held in the stores. The bin card is kept in the warehouse with the physical stock.

B. ARRANGING COMMODITIES

1. Organize the stock into different sections for different categories of supplies, for example, drugs, dressings, instruments, medical stationery, equipment and spare parts, laboratory supplies, disinfectants. For details see chapter on Inventory Management.

2. Clearly label each section of the store, allocate each item to a specific place and label the position of the item on the shelf so that it is easy to read.

Arranging the storeroom and shelves:

1. If using pallets, stack cartons on pallets-

    i. At least 10 cm (4 inches) off the floor

    ii. At least 30 cm (1 foot) away from the walls and other stacks

    iii. No more than 2.5 m (8 feet) high (general rule).

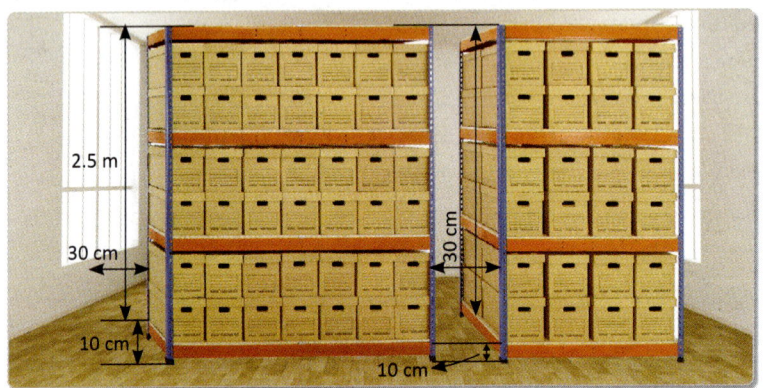

Arrangement of the storeroom and shelves

2. For all storage

All materials after inspection should be stored in the designated locations. Always materials should be stacked properly.

    i. Follow the manufacturer or shipper's directions when stacking, and follow labels for storage conditions.

    ii. Place liquid products on the lower shelves or on bottom of stacks.

    iii. Store products that require cold storage in appropriate temperature controlled zones.

    iv. Store high security/high value products in appropriate security zones.

    v. Store high alert/LASA drugs physically apart to avoid mix up. Use auxilliary labels to identify these.

    vi. Separate damaged or expired products from the usable stock without delay with proper label (as below), and dispose off using established disposal procedures (see section on Waste Management).

    vii. Arrange cartons so that arrows point up and identification labels, expiry dates, and manufacturing dates are visible. If this is not possible, write the product name and expiry date clearly on the visible side.

3. Preventing expiry of drugs at the health facility level

FEFO (First Expiry First Out) is a way of organizing, handling and priortization of moving of medicines. Material requirement are serviced in the order of items with the earlier date of consumption regardless of the date of entry or acquisition.

i. Always store all commodities in a manner that facilitates FEFO policy for stock management.

ii. The expiry date is one important assurance of drug quality. Rotate stock according to the expiry date using the FEFO First-In First-Out (FIFO) rules to have access to medicines with shortest expiry date first, put these in front of the shelves.

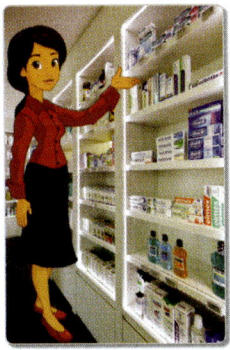 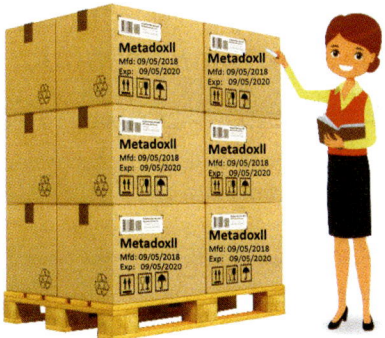

Stock rotation   FEFO policy

Stock with longer expiry date should be placed behind those with shorter dates.

iii. Use the FIFO rule for items without expiry date and mark those with the date of receipt.

iv. Put a red star or a similar mark on the labels of all items that have an expiry date within the current year. The dispensing pharmacist to check again the expiry date while indenting from the store.

v. Pharmacist in the dispensing counter to check again to ensure that no expired medicine are lying at the pharmacy and a register of expiring date is maintained.

vi. Have consumers check the expiry date themselves whenever possible.

vii. Details of the drugs with quantity in stock and date of expiry should be provided at least six months before the due date of expiry to the Doctors/Medical Officers to enable consumption of such drugs. This list should be updated every month and should be duly acknowledge by the in-charge concerned.

viii. The periodicity of this inspection/check should be once every month and should be duly certified in the drug expiry register by the designated personnel and should be physically checked that there is no discrepancy between the stock register and physical stock as per bin card.

ix. Ensure that out-of-date stock procedure is followed by clearly marking them in Black and segregating them from in date stock, until arrangements can be made to have the out-of-date stock destroyed.

x. Non-usable and expired medication should be taken off the shelf and should be stored in a separate, secure area under the control of the pharmacy until final disposal to avoid a chance of reaching consumers.

xi. Internal transfer/inter-inventory mechanism for excess stock: It is important that drugs are not allowed to expire in the health facility because of changes in disease pattern or for any other reasons. Items that can be used elsewhere should be transferred immediately from one health facility to another without including the central store for subsequent redistribution through proper indents. Excess stock should normally be transferred at least 3 months before expiry of the item.

xii. Detailed list of drugs due to be expired, with quantity available is to be shared with other hospitals/all health centre in their respective Health facility (HF)/district and the office of the in-charge concerned, through mail for effective circulation.

xiii. Expired stock must be disposed as per applicable Bio Medical Waste (BMW) Management Rules. For details see chapter on Handling of Expired or Damaged Stock and their Safe Disposal.

II. MONITORING PRODUCT QUALITY

A. INDICATORS OF QUALITY PROBLEMS

1. Products of different types show damage in different ways. Some indicators you can use to detect damage are:

Indicators of Quality Problems

All products

Quality of label design/colour and variations in colour combination in case of 2-colour gelatine capsules.

Missing, incomplete, or unreadable label(s)

Non-uniformity in packing methodology

Level of liquid preparation in bottle packings.

Tab/cap identical in size, shape and colour

Broken or ripped packaging (vials, bottles, boxes, etc.)

Liquids

Discolouration

Cloudiness

Sediment

Broken seal or bottle

Cracks in ampoule, bottle, or vial

Dampness or moisture in the packing

Light-sensitive products (such as x-ray film)

Torn or ripped packaging

Latex products

Dry

Brittle

Cracked

Lubricated latex products

Sticky packaging

Discoloured product or lubricant

Stained packaging

Leakage or the lubricant (moist or damp packaging)

Pills (tablets)

Discolouration

Crumbled pills

Missing pills (from blister pack)

Stickiness (especially coated tablets)

Unusual smell

Non-identical (scoring, lettering, numbering) tablet markings

Spots, pits, chips, breaks, uneven edges, cracks, embedded or adherent foreign matter

Injectables

Liquid does not return to suspension after shaking

Specks/foreign particles in dry solids for use in injections

Sterile products (including IUDs)

Torn or ripped packaging

Missing parts

Broken or bent parts

Moisture inside the packaging

Stained packaging

Capsules

Discolouration

Stickiness

Crushed capsules

No empty capsules

Tubes

Sticky tube(s)

Leaking contents

Perforations or holes in the tube

Foil packs

Perforation(s) in packaging

Chemical reagents

Discolouration

2. Need for laboratory testing should be carefully assessed.

3. If problem with quality are detectable on visual inspection (as above) then it does not require a laboratory test. The matter should be reported to appropriate authorities.

4. Damaged products should never be issued to facilities or dispensed. If you are not sure if a product is damaged, check with someone who knows. Do not issue or dispense products that you suspect are damaged.

5. Report any defects and send the defective products back to the facility that issued, DTC, appropriate Drugs Control Authority.

B. HANDLING COMPLAINTS ABOUT PRODUCT QUALITY

1. DTC should monitor and analyze all reports of inadequate medicine quality. The problem may present in the following ways:

    i. Visual deterioration of the product as reported by health staff, for example discolouration, fragmentation, leakage, smell, etc.

    ii. Lack of therapeutic effect

    iii. Adverse Drug Reactions (ADRs)

2. Once a problem has been reported, it should be investigated to see, if some problem is in one of manufacture (including counterfeit), storage, distribution, administration or use. This may involve the following steps:

    i. Confirming the exact nature of the problem.

    ii. Visually inspecting the product, including the expiry date, the packaging and the labeling.

3. The expiry date is one important assurance of drug quality.

4. Analysis of the product. A product may be analyzed first using basic (less expensive) tests, which can screen out counterfeit medicines or those of very poor quality. If the product passes such a screen, but has been the subject of complaints about quality, it should be subjected to further full pharmacopoeial (more expensive) tests in a properly equipped laboratory (Preferably accredited laboratory).

5. Report to the national/state regulatory authority about drug products found to be of poor quality on receipt from the manufacturer or supplier.

6. Quality problems are likely to be more serious in medicines that are inherently unstable or have a narrow therapeutic index (narrow range for effective serum levels). These medicines are listed in box below. The same drug product produced by different manufacturers may have differences in bioavailability and therefore be non-bioequivalent. It is much harder to ensure bioequivalence between products where the drug has a narrow therapeutic index. An additional quality factor to consider in drug selection and management is the varying stability of different forms of oral medicines.

Stability of oral drugs in increasing order

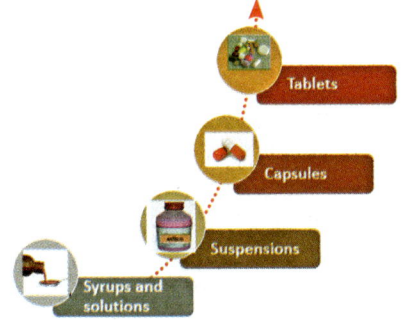

Generally speaking, solid forms are more stable than liquid forms, especially in tropical or humid conditions. Syrups and injections that are in powder form are more stable than those in liquid form.

Drugs with known potential bioavailability or stability problems

Bioavailability problems			Stability problems
aminophylline	furosemide	nitrofurantoin	acetylsalicylic acid tablets
ampicillin	glibenclamide	oestrogens	amoxicillin tablets
carbamazepine	glyceryl trinitrate	phenytoin	ampicillin tablets
chloramphenicol	griseofulvin	prednisolone	penicillin V tablets
chloroquine	hydrochlorothiazide	quinidine	retinol tablets
chlorpromazine	iron sulfate	rifampicin	paracetamol liquid
digitoxin	isosorbide dinitrate	spironolactone	penicillin V suspension
dehydroergotamine	levodopa	theophylline	ergometrine injection
ergotamine	methotrexate	L-thyroxine	methylergometrine injection
erythromycin	methyldopa	warfarin	

C. GUIDELINES FOR SENDING SAMPLES FOR QUALITY ASSURANCE TESTING

Quality assurance is the management activity required to ensure that the drug that reaches the patient is safe, effective and acceptable to the patient.

1. **If resources are limited, prioritize for quality assurance activities according to budget available and target sampling to products that**
   i. Have the greatest potential for bioavailability and stability problems
   ii. Are from new suppliers
   iii. Have been the source of complaints

2. **Sampling frequency**
   i. Upon arrival, laboratory testing of batch samples may be undertaken routinely or "by exception" depending on the policy. Testing "by exception" means that analyses are done only when a supplier or a particular drug product is a suspect.
   ii. With new suppliers for the first three deliveries their products should be sampled with greater frequency. Sampling from well established suppliers may be done much less frequently, often only for at-risk products.

3. **Tests to be done** depend on the drug product and the reason for testing. Basic chemical analyses are done to verify the identity of the drug and to look for degradation, chemical contamination, or adulteration.
   i. A complete analysis of tablet and capsule forms includes tests for identity, potency, uniformity, disintegration and dissolution.
   ii. Microbiological methods include sterility tests for injectable drugs and eye preparations and microbiological assays for antibiotics and vitamins.
   iii. Pharmacological tests include pyrogen test, toxicity test, hormone assays and tests to determine the bioavailability of selected drug products.

4. **Selection of laboratories for quality testing**
   i. Select from National List of Approved Testing Laboratories by CDSCO (http://cdsco.nic.in/writereaddata/ListapprovedtestingLaboratories.docx) or laboratories that are accredited by the National Accreditation Bureau for Testing and Calibration (NABL).

The lab should have the capacity and capability to issue test reports promptly. Preferably a panel of 4-5 laboratories for each drug should be set-up. To ensure reliability of test reports, the working of the selected laboratories should be validated by sending samples to more than one of such selected laboratories. To keep the cost of testing within acceptable range such samples may be required to be tested for specified tests. The reproducibility of results should also be compared.

ii. Track record of the performance of the each selected testing laboratory should be maintained for assessment of the quality of work. Suitable records for each activity must be available and inspected by a duly authorized person.

iii. **Steps involved in sending samples for testing:**

    a. Drawing of samples: Draw representative sample from the batch. Approximately for tablets -50 tablets; Ampoules and vials - 20-50 ampoules/vials; IV fluids 8-10 bottles. For details of the quantities of the drug required for test on tablets, capsules and injections see list of Central Drugs Laboratory, Kolkata. If an item requires special scrutiny further sample will be required, in addition, to the quantity stated in the list.

    b. Coding of samples: Immediately after receipt of the medicines from the supplier the material must be kept in safe custody under the control of the person duly notified for the purpose.

    c. Remove label to hide identity and origin of the medicine viz. in case of ampoules and injections remove label; for tablets and capsules remove from strips and pack the same in a bottle or test tube duly sealed.

    d. Assign specific code number by the in-charge of the stores. This specific code number should not be known to anyone except the duly notified person in-charge.

NOTE: This exercise is not applicable in case of tablets/capsules/ ampoules or other preparations where either name of the medicine or of the manufacturer is imprinted or the product has any sign/logo indicative of its origin.

5. **Dispatch of sample**

    i. The sample as well as the outer cover should be properly sealed along with a covering letter clearly mentioning – for test and report in accordance with Indian Pharmacopoeia or any other pharmacopoeia as specified by manufacturer or any one or more of the tests specified.

    ii. In case the drug is suspected to be spurious and quick report is required, the covering note should mention – for urgent test and urgent report on the specified test(s) e.g., identification and assay of the drug.

6. **Receipt and decoding of the sample on receipt of a report**

    • It should be done in the same manner as above.

    • Action to be taken as per terms and conditions of the agreement with the supplier. Also if the report is of NOT OF STANDARD QUALITY (NSQ), the Drugs Control Authority should be duly informed for statutory action.

    • If the report is not satisfactory or supplier challenges the test report, second sample should be sent to another approved laboratory.

7. The medicines remaining of the batch found to be NSQ should be segregated and no fresh issue should be made to patients or other health facilities.

8. Inform authorities for appropriate instructions. For details see section on Recall given in

Chapter on Good Dispensing Procedures. and Disposal of Expired or Damaged Stock and their Safe Disposal.

D. PREVENTING DAMAGING AND CONTAMINATION

1. **Physical damage:** Avoid crushing of products stored in bulk. Products should be stacked no more than 2.5 m (8 feet) high, as a general rule. Heavier or fragile items (such as those packaged in glass) should be placed in smaller stacks. Bind sharp edges or corners in the store with tape. Most important, ensure that nothing in the store can fall and injure members of the staff. Do not store products directly on floor.

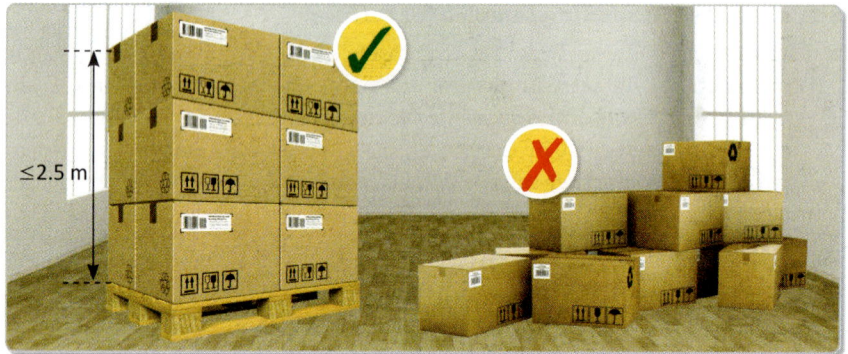

2. **Write and post the schedule and instructions** for cleaning the storeroom in multiple locations around the facility: Sweep and mop or scrub the floors of the storeroom regularly. Wipe down the shelves and products to remove dust and dirt. Disposal of garbage and other waste material should be done in a manner that avoids attracting pests. Store garbage in covered receptacles.

3. **Infrastructure:** Ensure the storeroom has easy access to a water outlet for cleaning. If no running water is available, set up a system using, for example, several 55 gallon drums on an elevated platform connected to pipes running into the store. Refill the drums regularly. When rehabilitating an existing storage facility or constructing a new structure, install water outlets in several locations inside the structure so that water is easily available from any location in the storeroom.

4. **Cleaning materials:** Keep a budget for buying cleaning materials. Use industrial detergents when possible, particularly for larger facilities. Try to use locally available detergents, particularly for smaller or more remote facilities. Clean with chlorine bleach regularly (once a month, for example).

5. **Outside the facility:** Burn garden rubbish and cardboard cartons, etc., only when garbage collection is not available. Use the necessary precautions to keep the fire under control, and do not burn materials close to the building. Make sure the wind is not blowing toward the building.

III. ROUTINE WAREHOUSE OR STOREROOM MANAGEMENT TASKS

The responsible pharmacist must ensure that all areas where medicines are stored are of acceptable standard. Specific tasks may differ based on locally established guidelines, procedures, and regulations, or the level in the system (e.g., health facility, district, region, or central).

1. **Daily**
   i. Monitor storage conditions.
   ii. Clean receiving, storage, packing, and shipping areas.

   iii.   Sweep or scrub floors.

   iv.   Remove garbage.

   v.   Clean bins, shelves, and cupboards, if needed.

   vi.   Ensure that aisles are clear.

   vii.   Ensure adequate ventilation and cooling.

   viii.   Ensure that products are protected from direct sunlight.

   ix.   Monitor store security and safety.

   x.   Check the store roof for leaks, especially during the rainy season and during or after a storm.

   xi.   Monitor product quality (visually inspect commodities and check expiration dates).

   xii.   Ensure that products are stacked correctly (are the lower cartons being crushed?).

2. Daily/Weekly

   i.   Update stock records[15] and maintain files.

   ii.   If cycle counting, conduct physical inventory and update stock-keeping records.

   iii.   Monitor stock levels, stock quantities, and safety stocks.

   iv.   Submit emergency order (as needed, using local guidelines).

   v.   Update back-up file for computerized inventory control records.

   vi.   Update bin cards.

   vii.   Separate expired stocks and move to secure area.

3. Monthly

   i.   Conduct physical inventory[16] or cycle count, and update stock-keeping records.

   ii.   Run generator to ensure the system is working correctly; check the level of fuel and add fuel, if needed.

   iii.   Check for signs of rodents, insects, or roof leaks.

   iv.   Inspect the storage structure for damage, including the walls, floors, roof, windows, and doors.

4. Every 3 months (quarterly)

   i.   Conduct physical inventory or cycle count (for details see inventory management), and update stock-keeping records to ensure that:

      a.   Medicines and scheduled substances are stored in accordance with the pharmaceutical manufacturer's requirements;

      b.   No out-dated or obsolete medicines are stocked;

      c.   Most medicines can be kept at uncontrolled room temperature. If there are no special instructions, normal storage conditions apply i.e., store in a dry , clean, well-ventilated premises at temperature of +15-25°C; max 30°C.

---

15 **Stock records**: A generic term that applies to bin cards, Kardex records, stock ledgers, and computer files. These provide basic information for inventory management providing all transactions for an item, including receipts, issues, orders placed, orders received, and stock losses.

16 **Stock count/physical inventory**: The process of inventory taking, in which a physical count is made of all items in inventory and compared with the written record.

d. Less stable medicines and injectables are stored in specific conditions as per manufacturer's instructions. Shelf life of some injectables are less stable (such as adrenaline, injectable preparations in solutions, some suppositories, creams, ointments, x-ray films) since they are particularly unstable at uncontrolled temperature. many injections need to be protected from light as well as from heat. Medicines requiring special environmental conditions are properly stored; and stock levels are appropriate;

e. Inflammable substances are stored separately and in an appropriate manner; and

f. Disinfectants and preparations for external use are stored separately from medicines for internal use.

ii. Visually inspect fire extinguishers to ensure that pressures are maintained and extinguishers are ready for use.

5. Tasks according to reorder interval and reporting schedule (usually monthly or quarterly)

i. Assess stock situation. Minimum and maximum stock/re-order level (for details see Quantification of medical Supplies);

ii. Stock control accounting for pharmaceutical products, received into and removed from stock;

iii. Identification and proper disposal of outdated, deteriorated, recalled or obsolete pharmaceutical products and the timely return of items for credit using established procedures to dispose of expired or damaged products;

iv. Recording of orders, usage as well as financial data for analysis, interpretation and planning by pharmacists, the drugs and therapeutics committee and pharmaceutical services.

v. Complete and submit requisition form (indent or "pull" systems).

vi. Determine issue quantity and issue products ("push" system).

vii. Store products using correct procedures; rearrange commodities to facilitate the first-to-expire, first-out (FEFO) policy (see section on receiving and arranging products).

viii. Complete required reporting and documentation.

6. Every 6 months

i. Conduct fire drills and review fire safety procedures.

ii. Inspect trees near the medical store and cut down or trim any tree with weak branches.

7. Every 12 months

i. Service fire extinguishers and smoke detectors.

ii. Conduct complete physical inventory and update stock-keeping records.

iii. Reassess maximum/minimum stock levels, and adjust, if needed.

IV. ENVIRONMENT CONTROL

Generally, medicines should be stored in their original container in a cool, dry and secure place. The stability/effectiveness of some medicines depends on storing them at the correct temperature, humidity, light, etc.

1. **Humidity:** When product label say "protect from moisture," store the product in a space with no more than 60% relative humidity. To reduce the effects of humidity consider-

i. **Ventilation:** Open the windows or air vents of the storeroom to allow air circulation. Ensure all windows have screens to keep out insects and birds, and either have bars or are not open wide enough for anyone to climb in. Put boxes on pallets and ensure there is space between pallets and the walls of the storeroom. Do not place products directly on floor.

ii. **Packaging:** Secure all lids. Never open a new container unless necessary.

iii. **Circulation:** Use a fan to circulate fresh (outside) air. In bigger storerooms you may need a ceiling fan. Standing fans are more useful in smaller storerooms. This requires electricity and some maintenance.

iv. **Air conditioners:** If possible, use an air conditioner. This is costly, depends on a constant supply of electricity, and requires regular maintenance. Depending on climatic conditions, a dehumidifier may be a less costly option. However, they also need a constant supply of electricity and require regular attention to empty the water containers.

2. **Sunlight:** Some health products are photosensitive and will be damaged if exposed to light. These include multiple vitamins, furosemide, chlorpheniramine maleate, hydrocortisone, latex products (such as male condoms), and x-ray film.

   To protect products from sunlight-

   i. Shade the windows or use curtains, if they are in direct sunlight.

   ii. Keep products in cartons.

   iii. Do not store or pack products in direct sunlight.

   iv. Use opaque plastic or dark glass bottles for products that require them.

   v. Maintain trees on the premises around the facility to help provide shade, but check them regularly to ensure that there aren't any branches that can damage the facilities.

3. **Heat:** Remember that heat will affect many products. It melts ointments and creams and causes other products to become useless. In hot climate, avoid storing pharmaceuticals next to poorly insulated external walls that are exposed to solar radiation. Such walls absorb and transmit heat, and internal surface temperature may rise substantially above the general internal air temperature at certain times of the day. Place shelving or pallets at least 0.6 meters away from external walls, or use the building perimeter for storage of items that are not heat sensitive. Following the guidelines listed earlier for protecting products from humidity and sunlight will also help protect products from heat.

4. **Monitoring:** Consistently monitor the temperature of the different areas within the storeroom.

   i. Keep thermometers in various places for monitoring (see section on monitoring temperature). But, even if you do not have thermometers, you can still monitor the heat. If you feel hot, your products are probably hot, too.

   ii. Keep the storeroom well ventilated (see section on humidity). For better ventilation, store boxes on pallets and leave room between rows and stacked boxes (see section on arranging products).

   iii. Keep direct sunlight out of storeroom.

   iv. Under ideal conditions, rooms with multiple refrigerators and/or freezers should have air conditioning. Refrigerators and freezers generate large amounts of heat, which can damage the equipment over time.

   v. If it is not possible to have air conditioning, install fans around the equipment to increase airflow. If installing fans, remember to place the fans so that air also flows in the spaces behind the refrigerators.

vi.   Ideally, larger facilities should have a cold room rather than numerous refrigerators.

5. **Power supply**

Arrange for a solar panel generator or alternative supply of electricity for cold rooms and refrigerators if the main source of electricity is not reliable. If the generator is not solar-powered, maintain a stock of fuel sufficient to run the generator for at least a few days (see section on storing flammables). Run the generator on a regular basis (at least once a month) to ensure the system is working properly. Larger facilities may want to contract out the maintenance of the generator and electrical system.

A. COMMON TERMS USED FOR STORAGE CONDITIONS

Indian Pharmacopoeia describes conditions for storage of some official substances which are likely to deteriorate, if not stored properly. The following terms related to temperature and medical supplies are used commonly. It is important to follow the manufacturer's recommended storage conditions for all products. The terms used under definite meanings of the pharmacopoeia are:

Store frozen: Some products, such as certain vaccines, need to be transported within a cold chain and stored at -20°C. Frozen storage is normally for longer-term storage at higher-level facilities.

Do not freeze or do not store over 8°C: To be kept in refrigerator (from +2°C to +8°C but not in the freezer chamber).

Keep Cold: Store at any temperature NOT exceeding 8°C and usually between 2°C and 8°C but must not be frozen. These are usually kept in the first and second part of the refrigerator (never the freezer).

This temperature is appropriate for storing vaccines for a short period of time. A refrigerator is a cold place in which the temperature is maintained thermostatically between 2°C and 8°C.

Keep cool: Store at 8°- 25°C. An article for which storage in a cool place is directed, may, alternatively, be stored in a refrigerator (at temperature between 2°C and 8°C), unless otherwise specified in the individual product monograph.

Store at room temperature or do not store over 30°C: Store at 15°-30°C

Store at ambient temperature: Store at the surrounding temperature. This term is not widely used due to significant variation in ambient temperatures. It means "room temperature" or normal storage conditions, which means storage in a dry, clean, well-ventilated area at room temperatures 15° to 25°C or up to 30°C, depending on climatic conditions.

Protect from moisture: To be stored in normal humidity at room temperature (Relative Humidity less than 60%).

Protect from light: To be stored in a light-resistant cupboard/drawer; to be provided by the manufacturer in a light-resistant container.

Standard storage temperatures description	Temperature range
Frozen	-20°C to -10°C
Store in a refrigerator/Cold (Vaccine, serum, antibiotics, hormones, vitamins & minerals)	2°C to 8°C
Store in a Cool place	8°C to 25°C (....by Air conditioner)
Room temperature or Protect from excess heat	8°C to 30°C (not to exceed 30°C) depending on local conditions
Controlled room temperature	20°C to 25°C

Periodic checking of Temperature and Humidity

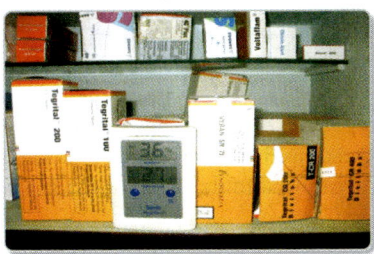

✓ Use max/min thermometer
✓ Probe should be placed in the centre of refrigerator
✓ Temperature should be recorded at least once a day
✓ Reset daily
✓ Calibrate as recommended
✓ Take immediate action, if temperature is outside recommended range

Temperature Monitoring Devices

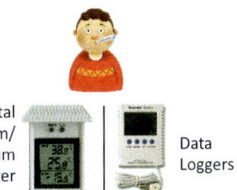

Digital Maximum/ Minimum thermometer

Data Loggers

B. COLD STORAGE OF PHARMACEUTICALS AND VACCINES

Cold chain[17] is the vital link in the potency and efficacy of the thermo labile products and immunization. *To maintain the potency of these products a safe zone of temperature is mandatory.*

1. Thermo labile medicines/biologicals/sera/vaccines must be kept in a refrigerator. Dedicated refrigerator must be used for pharmaceuticals/vaccines. Standard domestic refrigerators are not suitable for storing medicinal products requiring 2°C- 8°C storage, as it is difficult to maintain narrow temperature range required for the storage of such products due to minimal air circulation. Frequent opening and closing of the refrigerator door causes additional temperature fluctuations and the risk of products getting freezed particularly, if they come into contact with the chiller plate or coil at the back of the refrigerator.

2. A dedicated stand-alone pharmaceutical refrigerator, or units that only freeze or refrigerate are preferred for storage of thermolabile products/sera/vaccines with uninterrupted electrical supply and back up facilities should be available in the event of refrigerator failing. Frost-free or automatic defrost cycle refrigerators are preferred.

3. Never store food or beverages inside the vaccine refrigerator or freezer as this practice results in frequent opening of the storage unit door and greater chance for temperature instability and excessive exposure to light. It may also result in spills and contamination inside the compartment.

4. Do not store medications and other biologic products, if possible inside the vaccine storage unit. If there is no other choice, store these products below the vaccines on a different shelf to prevent contamination of the vaccines should the other products spill, and to reduce the likelihood of medication error.

5. Keep the refrigerator in the coldest room in the health facility. The refrigerator must be inside the dispensary or clinic and should be readily accessible to the pharmacist. The room should be well-ventilated and the refrigerator kept away from sunlight, heat and draughts. Draughts can blow out the flame in kerosene and gas refrigerators. Leave at least 20cm between the refrigerator, the wall and other equipment to allow hot air to escape from the back of the refrigerator. Make sure the refrigerator is on a firm, level base. If it has adjustable feet, adjust these by hand. If not, level the refrigerator by placing pieces of cardboard under each corner.

6. The size of the refrigerator must enable the pharmacist to keep the necessary stock in an organized manner. The size must therefore, prevent overloading of the refrigerator at any time (see also section on Temperature Monitoring).

7. Temperature-controlled storage areas must be equipped with temperature recorders.

8. Written procedures must be available detailing the actions to be taken in the event of a temperature violation.

---

17. A cold chain is a temperature-controlled supply chain from the point of production, during storage and distribution to the point of use.

C. STORAGE PRINCIPLES FOR THERMOLABILE PRODUCTS

It is important to store medicines properly and in accordance with any instructions given on the medicine label. The stability/effectiveness of some medicines depends on storing them at the correct temperature, for example, those medicines requiring refrigeration. These medicines requiring refrigeration need extra care and precaution, i.e. storage between the ranges of 2°C-8°C. It is necessary to ensure that the narrow temperature range required for the storage of such products has been maintained and that appropriate records are in place to demonstrate this are maintained at the pharmacy.

1. ***During transit and receiving:*** These products must be transported, handled and stored in a manner that mitigates the risk of exposure to temperatures outside labelled storage conditions. While receiving medicines which required controlled conditions (for example, temperature, relative humidity, light, etc.) during transit, examine the shipment upon reception, to ensure the conditions have been met and record the results. These products should be promptly transferred to the appropriate, environmentally controlled storage area.

2. When dispensing medicines to patients which require refrigeration, the pharmacists should give them information about suitable storage and transport of their medicines at home. Insulin is one of the commonly used thermolabile medicines is described in detail as below:

Special Handling Conditions for Insulin

Insulin must never be exposed to a temperature greater than +8°C or less than +2°C, as they can become inactive, or worse, in the event of significant and/or prolonged exposure, may also become toxic. Considering the low quantity of product that the insulin vials/pens contain, if exposed to an average room temperature of +20°C even for 3 minutes their increase in temperature is extremely fast to reach temperature of +8°C.

1. Receiving insulin from Distributors

    i.   For transportation of insulin from distributor to health facility/pharmacy, check that insulin is supplied in a rigid box with sensors and temperature logger for recording temperature within the box (temperature of 2-8°C should be maintained inside the box) at the time of supply.

    ii. Upon arrival from distributor transfer insulin immediately to refrigerator at 2-8°C. NEVER freeze or NEVER keep directly on ice.

2. Dispensing Insulin, from the pharmacy to the patients' refrigerator, and its storage

    Insulin needs to be dispensed with very clear instructions to the patient on how it should be transported to home and subsequently used as below:

    i.   Insulin should be transported without undue shaking and exposure to high (> 32 °C) or low (below 0 °C) temperature environments.

    ii. Insulin should be supplied in an insulated bag or cooling pouch to keep the insulin cold until patient reaches home (as shown). Insulated pouch and eutectic gel, which acts as the cold source (stored at +5 °C), maintains correct temperature for up to 1 hour (based on the conditions defined on the label).

    iii. Do NOT place insulin directly among ice cubes or strap insulin directly on a frozen ice pack as it may result in temperatures lower than the recommended 2°C. Allow sweating/conditioning of the ice packs (droplets appear on surface of ice pack) before putting insulin pack on the ice pack. Also do not transport insulin immersed in water as it destroys the labels on the insulin vials.

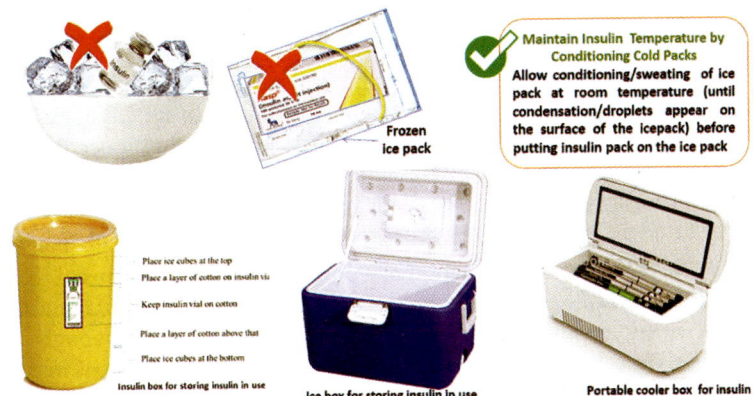

Maintain Insulin Temperature by Conditioning Cold Packs
Allow conditioning/sweating of ice pack at room temperature (until condensation/droplets appear on the surface of the icepack) before putting insulin pack on the ice pack

Frozen ice pack

Place ice cubes at the top
Place a layer of cotton on insulin via
Keep insulin vial on cotton
Place a layer of cotton above that
Place ice cubes at the bottom

Insulin box for storing insulin in use

Ice box for storing insulin in use

Portable cooler box for insulin

iv. ***Conditioning of Ice pack:*** Exposure to frozen ice pack can damage insulin. To avoid vaccine damage by cold packs, it's important to condition the cold packs before using them to store or transport. Conditioning cold packs involves letting them defrost for a short time at room temperature before using them. Remove cold packs from the freezer one to two hours before using them with vaccine. When the edges of the cold packs begin to defrost, and notice that the packs are "sweating" (or have condensation/droplets on them), they are conditioned and safe to use.

v. During its transportation, do not expose the medicine to the sun or heat. Insulin should remain in its original packaging to protect it from sunlight.

3. Storage at home
    i. Insulin should be transferred immediately in refrigerator and stored at the recommended temperature of 2–8 °C at home.

    ii. Store the insulin in the middle of the refrigerator, never in the vegetable compartment or in the door as these sections of the refrigerator are not as cold.

    iii. Never put the insulin in the ice compartment, or the freezer.

    iv. Store insulin away from the walls of the refrigerator or any food present.

    v. Label different insulin products with different coloured marked pens. Cartridges and pens come in different colours to demarcate different formulations. Store different insulin products in different areas of the refrigerator.

    vi. Store unopened insulin in refrigerator. Insulin (vials, pen, cartridges) in use may be kept at room temperature (20-25°C), protected from sunlight for a maximum of 4 weeks after initial use and within the expiry date) in a clean plastic box. Write expiration date on vials when opened. Do not use opened pen devices past expiration.

    vii. Insulin should never be kept immersed under water. Immersing opened insulin vial/cartridge under water as it carries a high risk of contamination, leading to loss of potency and likelihood of causing injection abscesses.

4. Optimisation of Injection Technique
    i. Injection sites: The four safe areas for insulin injections are the sides of the thighs, the backs of the upper arms, the abdomen and the upper outer buttocks; inject 2.5 cm (one finger breadth) away from scars and 5 cm (two finger breadths) away from the umbilicus. Do not inject insulin in bruised, swollen, or tender skin.

    ii. Rotate sites of injection every day so that insulin is not injected in the same place more than once in a day to avoid bumps and scar tissue on the skin.

    iii. There is no need to swab the area, if injection site is clean. If the injection site is not clean,

clean with plain water. Swabbing with spirit-swabs is not recommended as it leaves the skin dry.

iv. Needle and syringe: Use the shortest available needles (4 mm for pen or 6 mm for insulin syringe) with no requirement for lifting of skin fold (pinching); if longer needles are used lifting of a skin fold is required. In obese patient may use 6 mm needle, however, lifting a skin fold is not necessary in obese patients. In very thin patients, pen injections are preferred; pinching using 6 mm needle may be required for injection. The lifted skin fold should be lifted up gently and not squeezed tightly to causes skin blanching or pain.

v. Injection procedure is the same whether a pen device or syringe is used to administer the insulin. Aim the needle perpendicularly at an angle of 90°. Avoid intramuscular injections especially with long-acting insulins, as it may result in severe hypoglycaemia. Do not excessively slant the needle as it results in sub-epidermal injection of insulin which leads to poor absorption and may cause "tattooing" of the skin and scarring.

vi. Inject the insulin slowly and steadily and leave the syringe in place for 5–30 seconds after injecting; ensured by counting from 0 to 5 or up to 30.

vii. If insulin tends to leak from the injection site, put some pressure on the injection site with a piece of cotton swab for a few seconds: DO NOT RUB.

viii. If bleeding occurs, apply a cotton swab with some little pressure for 30 seconds. This is usually sufficient. DO NOT RUB.

ix. Put back the needle and syringe in a safe hard container. Close the container, and keep it safely away from children.

x. If more than 50 units of insulin is to be injected, insulin dose may be split and administered in divided doses either at different times or using different sites for the same injection. Large volumes of insulin are associated with more insulin absorption variability.

xi. Not to reuse the needle if possible; otherwise limit the reuse when injections become more painful; but should not reuse needles more than 5 times. Carefully recap needle but do not bend/cut needles.

xii. Disposal of needles and syringes in puncture proof box (not to be filled more than 70% of its capacity); puncture-proof containers disposed of in the trash, and sharps container disposal at designated sites, where available.

5. Travelling with Insulin Precautions

   i. Carrying insulin while travelling in hot climates can be a challenge. Insulin may be packed in a tight polythene bag and kept inside a small thermos flask in a carry-on bag but do not put insulin directly on ice or a gel pack.

   ii. Do not keep insulin in a locked car or in the glove compartment by a pool, in direct sunlight, or on the beach. Temperature in closed vehicles may reach very high levels (above 32 °C), with loss of potency of insulin. Heat can also damage blood sugar monitor, strips, insulin pump, and other diabetes equipment.

   iii. When travelling by air, carry insulin supplies, along with a prescription, in cabin baggage or handbag. Luggage which is checked-in is stored in the aircraft's hold and may freeze: any insulin in this luggage may lose its potency.

   iv. Do not store insulin near extreme heat (above 32°C) or extreme cold sources (below 2°C).

D. TYPE OF REFRIGERATORS AND FREEZERS

1. Freezers and refrigerators for vaccine storage and handling are available in many different sizes, types (e.g., standalone versus combination), and grades (e.g., household, commercial, pharmaceutical and laboratory). Stand-alone freezers and refrigerators without freezers are usually recommended.

2. Some of the desired features of the refrigerators are:
    i.   Refrigerators incorporate specifically designed refrigeration systems, protecting vaccines from freezing
    ii.   Microprocessor controls assure precise temperature throughout the chamber
    iii. Easy to view control panel displays with alarm systems that have access to remote monitoring
    iv.   Forced air systems provide close top-to-bottom uniformity at all shelf and drawer levels
    v.   Reserve cooling for rapid temperature recovery following door openings
    vi.   Tolerance for high ambient temperature with high performance refrigeration systems and superior CFC free insulation
    vii. Refrigerators that open on the top are more efficient than vertical ones, because hot air rises while cold air falls.

3. Using the correct freezer and/or refrigerator can help prevent costly vaccine losses and the inadvertent administration of compromised vaccines.

4. Preferably there should be dedicated refrigerator for each patient care areas to store biologicals and vaccines.

5. Vaccines are stored in a dedicated stand-alone freezers and refrigerators without freezers (frost-free or automatic defrost cycle refrigerator preferable), with adequate storage space to accommodate maximum inventory of vaccine.

6. If using a combination freezer-refrigerator unit to store vaccines, care must be taken to ensure that the freezer is not so cold that the refrigerator temperature drops below the recommended temperature range. There should be separate temperature controls (thermostats) for the freezer and refrigerator compartments.

7. Any freezer or refrigerator used for vaccine storage should have its own exterior door that seals tightly and properly, as well as thermostat controls. It must be able to maintain the required temperature range throughout the year.

8. Special characteristics of vaccine refrigerators are:
    i.   Ice-lining Vaccine storage refrigerators (ILRs)[18]- are designed to operate in different climatic conditions and exhibit special characteristics. The internal refrigerator walls are lined with ice packs/tubes. This ensures that during power outages the vaccine is maintained at the recommended temperature for a specific period of time.
    ii.   ILRs are tested for temperature stability at ambient temperatures of 27°C, 32°C and 43°C in accredited laboratories to ensure that at field conditions the equipment will perform optimally. The three temperature zones are referred to as cold, temperate and hot zones - corresponding to the maximum temperatures above. ILRs have excellent temperature recovery qualities. Temperature recovery is the refrigerator's ability to return to its set operating temperature after being exposed to an elevated temperature. The frequency and duration of door openings will raise the internal temperature of the refrigerator and, depending on the temperature recovery properties and methods employed on the refrigerator, this may cause unsafe vaccine storage temperatures. The temperature recovery in an ILR is very different from domestic refrigerators. ILRs are controlled by high accuracy thermometer sensors with fast responses and any deviation from the pre-set temperature is sensed in a timely manner. For this reason ILRs do not need to accommodate large loads or contain water bottles to keep the refrigerator's thermal mass higher to ensure efficient temperature regulation.

9. There should be uninterrupted electricity supply or alternative back-up refrigerator available in the event of the storage refrigerator failing.

---

18 Ice lined refrigerators are top opening refrigerators and can hold the cold air inside better than a refrigerator with a front opening. It can keep vaccine safe with as little as 8 hours continuous electricity supply in a 24 hour period. The bottom of the refrigerator is the coldest place: DPT, DT, TT and BCG should not be kept directly on the floor.

10. **Size of Refrigerator:** Refrigerators should have adequate shelves and are not filled to more than 50% of their capacity and have a space on the sides between the items stored and the walls to allow air movement.

    i. Refrigerator is not over-packed and there should be enough space to position vaccines and diluents two to three inches from the unit walls, ceiling, floor, and door; that allows vaccines. Vaccines and diluents to be arranged in rows and allow space between them to promote air circulation and always have enough frozen icepack to transport items requiring cold storage in cold boxes and/or vaccine carriers. Use only icepack filled with water. Do not use icepacks pre-filled with other liquids, which are usually blue or green.

    ii. When ordering cold chain equipment, larger facilities should reassess the needs for icepacks and icepack freezer space.

    iii. If there is enough space, place a few plastic bottles of water in the refrigerator. This will help maintain the temperature for a longer period of time if the power is cut off.

11. **Placement and Routine Maintenance of Refrigerator**

    i. Good air circulation around a vaccine storage unit is essential for proper cooling functions.

    ii. A storage unit should be placed optimally in a well-ventilated room, out of direct sunlight and away from external walls.

    iii. Vaccines must be secured away from public access. Vaccine refrigerators should be equipped with a lockable door or the vaccine refrigerator should be stored in a room with a lockable door.

    iv. Allow for space on all sides and top and allow at least 4-5 inches between storage unit and a wall to allow for air circulation.

    v. Ensure unit stands level with at least 1 to 2 inches between bottom of unit and floor.

    vi. Do not block motor cover.

    vii. Limit the number of times the refrigerator is opened. Do not overfill the compartments. If air cannot circulate freely inside the refrigerator, the temperature will rise.

    viii. Check that each unit door is closed tightly every day before leaving.

    ix. Check door seal at least once every month.

E. STORAGE PRINCIPLES FOR VACCINES

1. Named trained designated person and deputy should have overall responsibility for ordering, receipt and care of thermolabile products/vaccines. Assign a primary vaccine coordinator who is responsible for ensuring that vaccines are stored and handled correctly at each facility. Designate at least one alternate (back-up) vaccine coordinator who can perform these responsibilities in the absence of the primary coordinator.

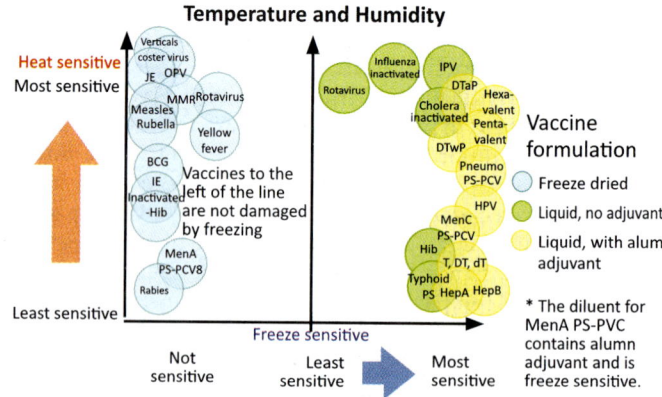

2. Vaccine stocks should be monitored regularly by the nominated staff members to avoid shortages, under or over-ordering or stockpiling especially ordering vaccines in multiple quantities or multi-dose vials.

3. Vaccine Stability Always protect the vaccine from heat & light.

MMR/MMRV, varicella, and zoster vaccines must be stored in a continuously frozen state in a freezer at 5°F (–15°C) or colder until administration. MMRV, varicella, and zoster removed from the freezer. Measles, mumps, and rubella vaccine (MMR) is routinely stored in the refrigerator, but it also can be stored in the freezer.

Live attenuated influenza vaccine (LAIV) and rotavirus vaccines are also live virus vaccines, but they should be stored in the refrigerator. Do not store these vaccines in the freezer.

Vaccines sensitive to both Heat and Cold

Inactivated vaccines are sensitive to both excessive heat and freezing. They should be stored in a refrigerator at 2° to 8°C, with a desired average temperature of 5°C. Exposure to temperatures outside this range results in decreased vaccine potency and increased risk of vaccine-preventable diseases. Inactivated vaccines may tolerate limited exposure to elevated temperatures, but they are cold sensitive and are damaged rapidly by freezing temperatures.

4. **Light sensitive vaccine** i.e. sensitive to strong light, sunlight, ultraviolet, fluorescents (neon) are:

- BCG   • MMR, MMRV
- Varicella
- Meningococcal C conjugate
- Most DTaP containing vaccines.

Exposure to light, causes loss of potency. These vaccines must be protected from light at all times. Therefore, store these vaccines at the appropriate temperatures in their boxes with the tops on until they are needed.

5. Vaccines should not be stored for longer than the specified storage period. All vaccines and diluents must be stored in the refrigerator for short term between 2°C and 8°C in a pharmacy that issues to the end-user or clinics. For long term storage at -20°C is preferred only for BCG, OPV, and measles/MMR. **Do not freeze other vaccines**.

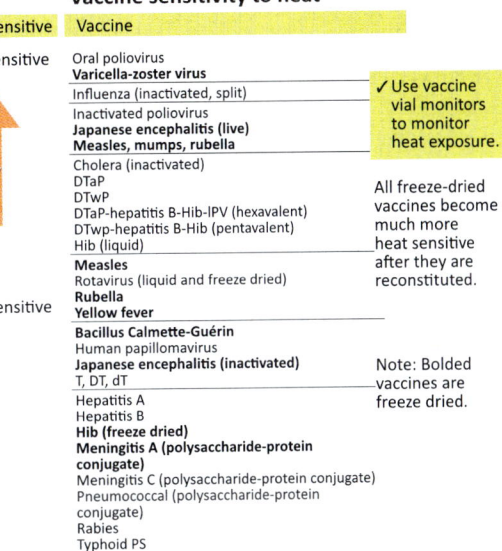

Vaccine sensitivity to heat

Heat sensitive	Vaccine	
Most sensitive	Oral poliovirus	
	Varicella-zoster virus	
	Influenza (inactivated, split)	✓ Use vaccine vial monitors to monitor heat exposure.
	Inactivated poliovirus	
	Japanese encephalitis (live)	
	Measles, mumps, rubella	
	Cholera (inactivated)	
	DTaP	All freeze-dried vaccines become much more heat sensitive after they are reconstituted.
	DTwP	
	DTaP-hepatitis B-Hib-IPV (hexavalent)	
	DTwp-hepatitis B-Hib (pentavalent)	
	Hib (liquid)	
	Measles	
	Rotavirus (liquid and freeze dried)	
	Rubella	
Least sensitive	**Yellow fever**	
	Bacillus Calmette-Guérin	
	Human papillomavirus	
	Japanese encephalitis (inactivated)	Note: Bolded vaccines are freeze dried.
	T, DT, dT	
	Hepatitis A	
	Hepatitis B	
	Hib (freeze dried)	
	Meningitis A (polysaccharide-protein conjugate)	
	Meningitis C (polysaccharide-protein conjugate)	
	Pneumococcal (polysaccharide-protein conjugate)	
	Rabies	
	Typhoid PS	

Vaccine sensitivity to freezing

Freeze sensitivity	Vaccine	
Most sensitive	DTaP	
	DTaP-hepatitis B-Hib-IPV (hexavalent)	**Cautions:**
	DTwP	✓ Never expose these vaccines to zero or subzero temperatures.
	DTwP-hepatitis B-Hib (pentavalent)	
	Hepatitis A	
	Hepatitis B	
	Human papillomavirus	✓ Avoid the use of ice for transport.
	Meningitis C (polysaccharide-protein conjugate)	
	Pneumococcal (polysaccharide-protein conjugate)	
	T, DT, dT	
	Cholera (inactivated)	* While the stability data for liquid rotavirus vaccines demonstrate some resistance to freezing, the temperature handling recommendations in the vaccine product insert should be followed.
	Influenza (inactivated, split)	
	Hib (liquid)	
Least sensitive	Inactivated poliovirus	
	Typhoid ps	
	Rotavirus (liquid)*	
These vaccines are not damaged by freezing.	Meningitis A (polysaccharide-protein conjugate)T	
	Yellow fever	
	Bacillus Calmette-Guérin	T The diluent for MenA PS-PCV contains alum adjuvant and is freeze-sensitive.
	Hib (freeze dried)	
	Japanese encephalitis (live and inactivated)	
	Measles	
	Measles, mumps, rubella	
	Oral poliovirus	Note: Bolded vaccines are freeze dried.
	Rabies	
	Rotavirus	
	Rubella	
	Varicella-zoster virus	

Adopted from Temperature Sensitivity of Vaccines March 2014. WHO https://www.who.int/immunization/programmes_systems/supply_chain/resources/VaccineStability_EN.pdf

6. Domestic refrigerator, ice lined refrigerator are used for short term storage and deep freezer for long term storage. Box below depicts potency & temperature for storage of vaccines.

Potency & temperature for storage of vaccines.

Vaccine	Temperature	Potency maintained for	Remarks
Oral Polio (OPV)	-20°C	1 year	Avoid repeated thawing
	4°C to 8°C	3 months	Keep on ice while using
Bacillus Calmette Guerine (BCG)	4°C to 8°C	1 year	Reconstituted vaccine, if not used within four hours must be discarded
Diphtheria, Pertussis, Tetanus (DPT)	4°C to 8°C	2 years	Must not be frozen
Diphtheria, Tetanus (DT)	4°C to 8°C	2 years	Must not be frozen
Measles	0°C to 2°C	2 years	Should be used immediately after reconstitution
Typhoid (TAB)	4°C to 8°C	8 months	Must not be frozen
Tetanus toxoid (TT)	4°C to 8°C	18 months	Must not be frozen. Unused portion must be discarded.
Hepatitis B	4°C to 8°C	4 years	Must not be frozen

7. If vaccines are stored in a domestic refrigerator, it should be used only for vaccine storage. Store DPT, DT, TT and BCG vaccines away from the inside walls or bottom of the ILR to avoid freezing. It is better to keep them in the basket provided in the ILR.

8. Vaccines must NOT be kept:
   i. In the baffle tray or door compartments of domestic refrigerators;
   ii. In such a way that they can come into contact with the evaporator plate i.e., not close to the back or top of the compartments.

9. Correct packing of vaccines and diluents in the refrigerator is vital if they are to be kept at safe temperatures. Vaccines must be stored in such a way that they cannot be confused with other thermo labile drugs.

10. Diluents should be at the same temperature as the vaccine at the point of use.

11. Only the designated diluents should be used for specific vaccines.

12. Repeated thawing should be avoided for all practical purposes.

13. When defrosting refrigerator, keep vaccines in thermocol box or vaccine carrier containing ice packs.

14. During vaccination session, if it is of long duration, vials of vaccines taken out of refrigerator should be kept in a cup containing ice.

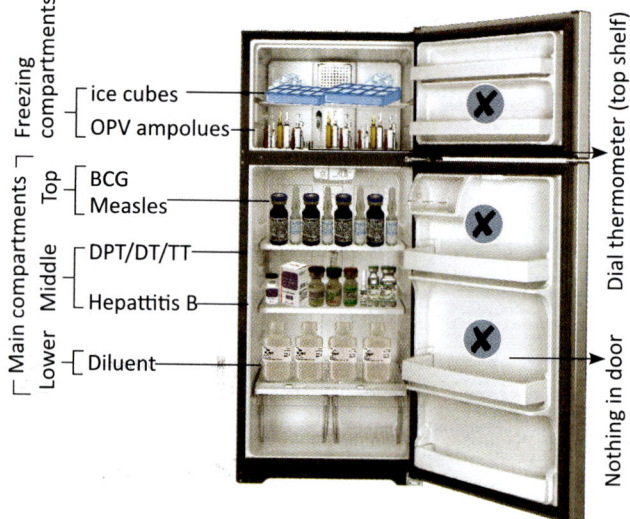

Refrigerator showing vaccines stored correctly in clinic setup

F. TESTING/AIDS FOR CHECKING APPROPRIATE STORAGE

Maintaining cold chain requires constant vigilance. Vaccine appearance is not a reliable indicator that vaccines have been stored under appropriate conditions. Some vaccines may show physical evidence that potency has been reduced when exposed to inappropriate storage conditions. This may appear as clumping in the solution that does not go away when the vial is shaken. Other vaccines may look normal when exposed to inappropriate storage conditions (see photos below). For example, inactivated vaccines exposed to freezing temperatures (i.e. 32°F [0°C] or colder) may not appear frozen and give no indication of reduced or lost potency.

1. Various aids can be used to monitor the temperature of vials, e.g. cold chain monitors (CCMs) and vaccine vial monitors (VVMs).

    i. Time temperature indicator known as a vaccine vial monitor (VVM) is absolutely vital as it allows health workers to know vaccine has not been exposed to excessive heat.

    ii. A vaccine vial monitor (VVM) is a label containing a heat sensitive material which is placed on a vaccine vial to register cumulative heat exposure over time. Such as polio and hepatitis B vaccine.

    iii. VVM colour change is a continuous process. The combined effects of time and temperature cause the inner square (active surface) of the VVM to darken gradually and irreversibly. A direct relationship exists between the rate of colour change and temperature:

        a. The lower the temperature, the slower the colour change.

        b. The higher the temperature, the faster the colour change.

Symbol	Explanation	Stage
✔	The inner square is lighter than the outer circle. If the expiry date has not passed, USE the vaccine.	I
✔	As time passes the inner square is still lighter than the outer circle. If the expiry date USE the vaccine.	II
✗	Discard point: the colour of the inner square matches that of the outer circle. DO NOT USE the vaccine.	III
✗	Beyond the discard point: inner square is darker than the outer circle. DO NOT USE the vaccine.	IV

    iv. Vaccines with darker circles (Stage II) must be selected for administration first. Do not use Stage III and IV vaccines.

    v. VVMs are located either on the label or on the top of the cap or on the top of the cap (vials) or on the neck of the ampoule so it is discarded by the time of reconstitution. Since freeze-dried vaccines must be discarded within six hours or at the end of the session whichever comes first, VVM can only be referred until the time of reconstitution.

2. **Shake Test:** The Shake Test will confirm whether DPT, DT, TT, Hepatitis B, Typhoid or Hib vaccines have been frozen. If a vaccine has never been frozen, the liquid will be smooth and cloudy immediately after shaking, and will have no or very little sediment 30 minutes after standing. When the vial is tilted the sediment will move.

If the vaccine has been frozen, granular particles (flocculation) will be seen on close inspection, and heavy sediment will be visible after standing for 30 minutes. This sediment will be less likely to move when the vial is tipped. Hepatitis B has very small flocculates when it has been frozen and the sedimentation test is the most reliable for judging, if it has been frozen. If a comparison is made between a vial known to be unfrozen and a suspect vial it is imperative that the two vials are from the same manufacturer and the same batch. **DO NOT USE SUCH VACCINE. SHAKE TEST IS NOT TO BE PERFORMED FOR OPV, MEASLES AND BCG VACCINES.**

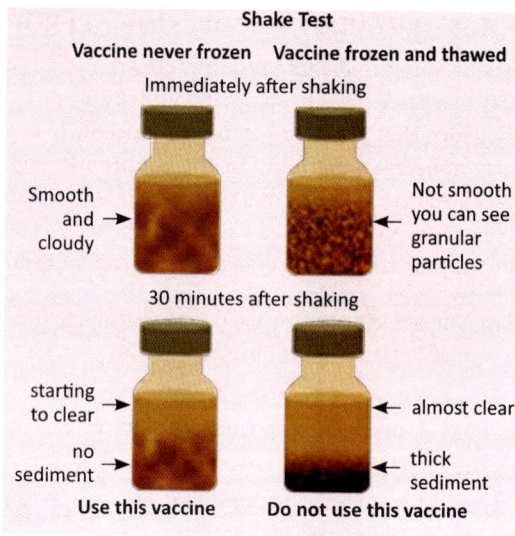

G. VACCINE STOCK MANAGEMENT

1. Check vaccine and diluent expiration dates a minimum of weekly.

2. Rotate stock so that vaccines and diluents with the first expiration dates are used first to avoid waste from expiration. If normal in appearance and stored adequately, not exposed to extremes of temperature, vaccine can be used: If the date on the label has a specific month, day, and year, the vaccine can be used through the end of that day. If the expiration date on the label is a month and year, the vaccine can be used through the last day of that month.

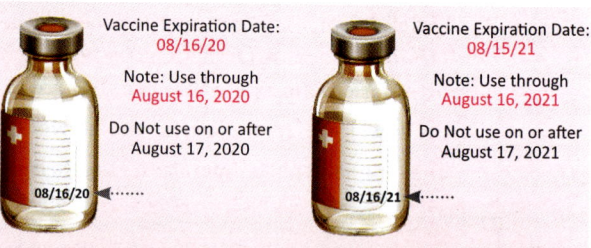

Check and arrange vaccines and diluent in storage unit according to expiration dates at least once each week and each time vaccines are delivered

3. Single-Dose Vials (SDV) are approved for use on a SINGLE person for a SINGLE procedure or injection. These singel dose vials typically lack an antimicrobial preservative. . Therefore, do NOT save or combine ("pool") leftover medication from these vials – harmful bacteria can grow and infect a patient/ resident. Discard after EVERY use.

4. Multi-Dose Vials (MDV) can be used for more than one person when aseptic technique is followed, but ideally used for only one person. Typically MDV contain an antimicrobial preservative to help limit growth of bacteria but have no impact on growth of bloodborne viruses. Discard when the beyond-use date or expiration date (see below) has been reached or any time the sterility of the vial is in question! If a multi-dose vial enters the immediate patient treatment area (e.g., patient's room), it should be dedicated for use by that person only and discarded immediately after use.

5. Vaccines deteriorate rapidly after they are opened. Mark each opened multidose vial with the date it was first opened with your initials.

6. Multidose vials (unopened) can be used through expiration date mentioned on vial as stated in manufacturer's product information. However, once reconstituted or opened should be used within time frame indicated by manufacturer or discarded as appropriate. For example, multidose vials of meningococcal vaccine should be discarded if not used within 35 days after reconstitution, even if the expiration date printed on the vial by the manufacturer has not passed.

7.   Reconstituted vial

i.   Some multidose reconstituted vaccines vials should be used within a certain time frame after the first time a needle is inserted, i.e. after the vaccine is reconstituted. This time frame is called the "**beyond use date**" or BUD. The BUD is the date or time after which the vaccine should not be used. It may not be the same as the expiration date. Putting a date on opened or reconstituted vials helps manage vaccine inventory by identifying vials that should be used first.

MULTI- DOSE VIAL

Date opened _____
Expiry Date _____
Initials _____

Mention date of opening on reconstituted multidose vials or Beyond Use Date (BUD)

ii.   The BUD varies among vaccines and check for BUD and for the correct time frame (e.g. days, hours) the vaccine can be stored once the vial has been entered or has been reconstituted in the package insert. Label the vaccine with the correct BUD.

iii.   Whenever possible, use all the vaccine in one multidose vial before opening another vial. Similarly, use all the reconstituted vaccine in one vial before reconstituting another vial. This policy helps to reduce vaccine waste.

iv.   Follow safe injection practices - During the procedure use aseptic technique. Use a NEW needle and syringe for every injection. Use a new needle and syringe even when obtaining additional doses for the same person. Do not leave the needle in the vial septum, if using the vial for multiple uses. Clean your hands immediately before handling any medication. Disinfect the vial by wiping the rubber septum with alcohol.

H. VACCINE AND DILUENT STORAGE LOCATION AND POSITIONING

1.   Store vaccines away from walls, coils, cooling vents, top shelf, ceiling, storage unit door, floor, and back of unit.

2.   Vaccine should be placed with space between the vaccine and the compartment wall, and with space between each large box, block, or tray of vaccine to allow for cold air circulation around the vaccine. Adequate cold air circulation helps each vaccine to reach a consistent temperature throughout its mass and is necessary for the storage unit to maintain a consistent temperature inside the compartment.

3.   Packing any vaccine storage unit too tightly will affect the temperature.

4.   Do not store vaccines in the freezer or refrigerator door or vegetable or fruit crisper drawers.

5.   If the upper shelf must be used for vaccine storage, it would be best to place MMR on this shelf with water bottles placed close to the vent because MMR is not sensitive to freezing temperatures like the other refrigerated vaccines.

6.   Keep vaccines and diluents in original packaging with lids on to protect from light, e.g. live attenuated vaccines, and some inactivated vaccines.

7.   Always follow the manufacturer's guidance in the product information/package inserts for storage of vaccine and diluent.

8.   Diluents packaged separately from their corresponding vaccines can be stored at room temperature or in the refrigerator.

9. Diluents packaged with their vaccines should be stored in the refrigerator next to their vaccines.

10. Some diluents may contain vaccine antigen. **Never store diluents in the freezer**. Diluents may be stored in refrigerator door.

I. VACCINE PACKAGING

1. Vaccine products that have similar packaging (Look alike) should be stored in different locations to avoid confusion and medication errors, e.g. pediatric and adult versions of the same vaccine, storing them in different locations lessens the chance that someone will inadvertently choose the wrong vaccine.

2. Likewise, vaccines that have similar sounding names should be stored in different locations.

3. Do not store soundalike and look-alike vaccines next to each other, e.g. DTaP and Tdap vaccine and Hib and hepatitis B vaccines and use auxiliary labeling to idetify look-alike and sound-alike vaccines.

J. VACCINE LABELLING

1. Clearly label the location of each specific vaccine inside the storage unit.

2. Attach labels directly to the shelves on which the vaccines are sitting or label trays or containers according to the vaccines they contain.

3. Stack in rows with same type of vaccine and diluent. Label diluent to avoid inadvertent use of the wrong diluent when reconstituting a vaccine. Label diluents clearly, whether they are stored at room temperature or in the refrigerator.

4. Label the boxes of corresponding vaccines and diluents from the same manufacturer so that they will be used together to avoid confusion and helps to ensure that only the specific diluent provided by the manufacturer for each type of lyophilized (freeze-dried) vaccine is used. This is particularly important if two or more lyophilized vaccines using different diluents are stored together.

Vaccine Storage Do's and Don'ts

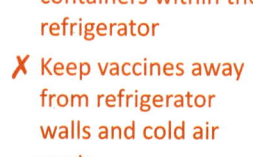

✗ No food or medical specimens

✗ Do not place refrigerator in direct sunlight or near heat source

✗ Do not remove vaccines from original boxes until ready to use

✗ Do not store vaccines in refrigerator doors or in solid plastic trays/ containers within the refrigerator

✗ Keep vaccines away from refrigerator walls and cold air vents

✓ Use a dedicated vaccine refrigerator – frost free, separate door

✓ Place vaccines in clearly labelled plastic mesh baskets

✓ Group vaccines by type (Paed, Adult, Adolescent)

✓ No more than 50% full

✓ Safeguard electricity supply

✓ Ensure back up facilities are available in the event of refrigerator failing

✓ Defrost/calibrate refrigerator regularly

5. Use uncovered storage containers to organize vaccines and diluents.

6. Place vaccines in clearly labelled plastic mesh baskets.

7. Group vaccines by type (Paediatric, Adult, Adolescent) and store paediatric and adult vaccines on different shelves.

8. Use labels with vaccine type, age, and gender indications or colour coding.

9. Store all opened and unopened vials of vaccine in their boxes inside the appropriate storage unit.

K. TEMPERATURE MONITORING

1. Temperature monitoring devices (TMD)

i.   Temperature monitoring device is an essential requirement for vaccine temperature monitoring. An accurate temperature history that reflects actual vaccine temperatures is critical for protecting vaccines.

ii. Many TMDs are available such as simple minimum/maximum thermometer, which only shows the coldest and warmest temperatures reached in a unit; digital data loggers (DDL) are continuous temperature recording devices, which offer a historical account of refrigerator temperatures.

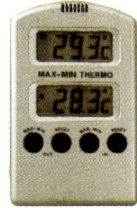 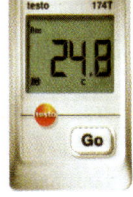 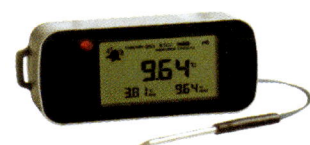

Digital maximum-minimum thermometers　　Data loggers　　Digital Data logger

Digital temperature monitoring devices

Unlike minimum/maximum thermometer, a DDL provides detailed information on all temperatures recorded at preset intervals.

• Use a DDL or other appropriate TMD for:
• Each vaccine storage unit
• Each transport unit (emergency or non-emergency)
• Have at least one backup TMD in case a primary device breaks or malfunctions.

iii. DDL with following features are preferred:
• Detachable probe that best reflects vaccine temperatures (e.g., a probe buffered with glycol, glass beads, sand, or Teflon®)
• Alarm for out-of-range temperatures
• Low-battery indicator
• Logging interval (or reading rate) that can be programmed by the user to measure and record temperatures at least every 30 minutes.

iv. Temperature monitoring devices need to be accurate. Use TMDs with a current and valid Certificate of Calibration Testing. Calibration testing should be done every one to two years or according to the manufacturer's suggested timeline.

v.   Do not use devices sold in hardware and appliance stores as they are designed to monitor temperatures for household food storage.

2. Refrigerator Temperature Record Chart

i.   The temperature of the refrigerator must be maintained between 2°C and 8°C.

ii. Temperature of ice lined refrigerators (ILRs)/Freezers/refrigerator used for storage of vaccines must be recorded **TWICE DAILY (morning and evening)**.

The sample of temperature record see below.

iii. The temperature chart earmarked for each equipment should be seen and signed by the officer-in-charge. These records should be checked during supervisory visits.

iv. A break in the cold chain is indicated, if temperature rises above +8°C or falls below +2°C in case of ILR & other refrigerators.

Sample refrigerator temperature record chart

v. Record the period of time for which all vaccines are exposed to temperatures above +8°C and DPT, DT and TT vaccines below 0°C.

vi. When an electricity disruption occurs, document the time and the maximum, minimum and current temperature inside of the non-functioning refrigerator in the Temperature Log Book.

vii. Do not allow the vaccine to remain in a non-functioning unit for an extended period of time.

L. VACCINE STORAGE TROUBLESHOOTING

1. In order to maintain the proper temperature ranges, the freezer and refrigerator units must be in good working condition and they must have uninterrupted power supply. Always have an alternative means of vaccine storage available. Give one person responsibility for the refrigerator, including storing vaccines, diluents and ice-packs, checking and recording the temperature, and maintaining the cold chain.

2. Make sure the health facility has a plan of what to do, if the refrigerator breaks down and that staff are trained to carry it out. Things which can be done to prevent problems are:

   i. Plug storage units directly into wall outlets.

   ii. Plug only one storage unit into an outlet. Do not use multi-outlet power strip.

   iii. Do not use power outlets with built-in circuit switchers.

   iv. Do not use power outlets that can be activated by a wall switch.

   v. Mark the plug clearly so the refrigerator is not unplugged or turned off accidentally.

   vi. Use plug guards or safety-lock plugs to prevent someone from inadvertently unplugging the unit. A temperature alarm system that will alert staff to after-hour temperature excursions.

   vii. Label circuit breakers by posting a warning sign near the electrical outlet, on storage units, and at the circuit breaker box. Warning signs should include emergency contact information.

viii.   Perform daily inspection of storage unit(s).

M. MAINTENANCE OF THE REFRIGERATOR

1. Daily checks

i.   Check the temperature every morning and evening. The temperature pattern will show if there are any faults or the refrigerator is not working efficiently.

ii.   Use max/min thermometer to find out the coldest and warmest refrigerator had been.

iii.   Always remember to reset your maximum-minimum thermometer (if applicable) after each recorded temperature.

iv.   Ensure placement of thermometer in the centre of refrigerator—away from door, near or against the walls, close to vents, floor.

v.   Check the freezer for ice build up.

vi.   Report faults to the maintenance officer immediately.

vii.   Calibrate using calibrated thermometers (with a certificate of calibration testing from an accredited laboratory). Calibrate every 1 to 2 years or as per manufacturer's instructions.

2. Monthly

i.   Clean once a month at least and remove and store vaccines in another functioning refrigerator to cold chain while cleaning

ii.   Defrost when there is more than 1 cm (¼ inch) of ice in the freezer compartment. While defrosting the refrigerator, transfer vaccines to an insulated vaccine container (for no longer than 3 hours) with icepacks and temperature monitoring device or transfer vaccines to another monitored refrigerator, and check the temperature regularly.

iii.   Perform refrigerator maintenance as required, including cleaning and dusting the back (including coils, top and sides) and ensuring the door is sealed tightly and properly (has adequate door seals and tight door hinges). Swab the inside of the cabinet with 70% ethanol while defrosting and keep the door open. Use water and detergent to clean the inside and outside of the refrigerator. Do not use abrasives or bleach, because these will leave grooves that allow micro-organisms to multiply. Dry all surfaces with a clean, soft, dry cloth.

iv.   Return vaccines, diluents and ice packs to their appropriate places. But, only put stock back in the refrigerator when the required temperature (0-8°C) has been reached. Do not restock vaccines immediately when refrigerator has been defrosted by setting the thermostat at the coldest setting. This can cause vaccines to freeze making them useless.

v.   Keep icepacks in the freezer compartment to use for transporting vaccines. In the case of a refrigerator malfunction or electricity disruption, icepacks can be put inside the refrigerator to keep the temperature from increasing. If power supply is off for any length of time, the refrigerator should not be opened till the time power supply is restored.

vi.   Follow the maintenance schedule and checks as advised by the manufacturer.

vii.   Oil the door fittings, locks and other moving parts. Check that the door is sealing correctly and, if necessary, change the door gasket. Check for visible damage, clean off patches of rust and repaint.

N. TEMPERATURE MAINTENANCE DURING TRANSPORT

Vaccines are damaged by heat wheher they are exposed to a lot of heat in a short time (e.g., cold chain equipment breakdown, delivery or outreach trips exceeding the container's cold life; Vehicle breakdown; parking vehicles in direct sunlight) or a small amount of heat over a long time (as a result of frequent opening of a refrigerator door).

1. An insulated container, temperature monitoring device and appropriate packaging material is used for:

    i.   Transporting vaccine;

    ii. Storing vaccine during immunization sessions/clinics;

    iii. Temporary storage of vaccine during equipment maintenance periods (e.g. when cleaning or defrosting refrigerator)

    iv. Emergency storage of vaccine (e.g. refrigerator malfunction or an electricity disruption).

2. Vaccines should be maintained within +2 °C to +8 °C inside properly packaged insulated containers (validated) during storage and transport.

3. **THE VIALS OF DPT, DT, AND TT VACCINES SHOULD NOT BE PLACED IN DIRECT CONTACT WITH FROZEN ICE PACKS.** The ice packs should be sufficient to give the container twice the length of cold life anticipated for a particular journey. For example: if a courier service guarantees to deliver a package within 24 hours that package must have a cold life of a minimum of 48 hours. *Never carry vaccines in a flask for an outreach place.* Vaccines which are naturally stored frozen (Polio), may be refrozen after transportation.

4. Vaccine carriers should be used for carrying small quantities of vaccines (16-20 vials) to the sub center or villages by health workers.

5. Insulated containers can maintain the required temperature for 3–4 hours; however, this is subject to environmental and physical conditions. Insulated containers are not adequate for the transport and/or storage of vaccines for prolonged periods as their cold life is limited. However, the external temperature, the number of times the insulated container is opened, the amount of vaccine that is being stored and the type of packaging material used may reduce the amount of time vaccines can be stored in the insulated container.

6. If vaccines are required to be stored and/or transported for more than 3–4 hours in the insulated container, the icepack(s) and/or gel pack(s) should be removed and replaced with a new set of conditioned frozen and/or refrigerated icepack(s) and/or gel/pack(s).

7. Ice and/or gel packs must be correctly conditioned before use. The risk of freezing vaccines increases if the icepacks/gel packs are not correctly conditioned.

8. During transportation of vaccines in an insulated container, continue to monitor temperatures during vaccine transport. However, the frequency of the checking and the recording of temperatures are dependent on the amount of time the vaccine is stored and transported in the insulated container.

9. Do not place insulated containers with vaccines in the trunk of a car.

10. Packing the vaccine carriers:

    i.   Confirm that there are no cracks in the walls of the vaccine carrier.

    ii. Take out the required number of ice packs from the deep freezer and wipe them dry.

    iii. Place fully frozen ice packs in the carrier and wait for few minutes for temperature to fall to less than 8° C.

iv. Wrap vaccine vials and ampoules in thick paper (say newspaper) before putting in polythene bag so as to prevent them from touching the ice packs. Place some packing material between vaccine and the ice packs to prevent them from touching the ice packs.

v. Ensure that some ice is present while conducting immunization sessions. However, with regard to VVM vaccine, it may be used till VVM is at stage I or II.

vi. Secure the lid tightly.

vii. If more than one vaccine carrier is being carried, keep the whole range of the vaccines required for the day's use in each carrier so that only one carrier is opened at a time.

   a. Keep the carrier in good condition when not in use: clean and dry the inside after every use.

   b. Use the shortest route to the health center and cover the distance quickly and safely.

   c. Transfer vaccines to the ILR/freezer IMMEDIATELY after arriving at the health center.

   d. Follow First –in-first –out (FIFO) and first to expire first to out (FEFO) rule.

   e. The sub center should not be provided more than their requirement. The vaccines should be returned to the PHC on the same day. All vaccines removed from the ILR/freezer must be used or returned to the ILR/freezer after the immunization session. If it is not possible to return the vaccines on the same day, they can be sent on the next day only if the ice packs/ice has not fully melted. Opened vials of the vaccines should be sent to PHC for discarding and not reused the next day.

   f. Vaccine that has been returned unused and unopened must be used during the following session, or failing this, during the third session. If it is not used even during the third session, discard it. Do not take the same vial of the vaccine out to the field more than THREE TIMES. If a vial of vaccine has been taken to the field third time, return it to the PHC after marking 'Discard'.

   g. If ice packs in the carrier still contain ice and to ensure that RETURNED vaccine is selected first, place these vials in a box in the ILR marked "returned". Put one rubber band for the first visit, and two if the vial was taken out twice.

   h. If the ice in the cold chain container is completely melted for less than one day:

   • Examine the VVM status on vial of OPV. NEVER USE OPV WITH VVM IN STAGE III AND IV (Discard it). If it is in stage I or II, look for the date of expiry. If it has not passed, it can be used.

   • Mark the remaining DPT, TT, measles and BCG vaccine, return to the ILR/freezer and use it during the next session.

   • If the ice in the cold chain container is completely melted for more than one day, throw away all vaccines.

   • Update records on vaccine use: keep record of the vaccines administered, batch numbers and expiry dates and vaccines returned to PHC.

   i. Check that DPT, DT or TT vaccines have not been frozen. If these have been frozen, DO NOT USE THEM. Confirm this by shake test described as above.

viii. VACCINES ARE NOT TO BE STORED AT THE SUB-CENTER LEVEL AND MUST BE SUPPLIED ON THE DAY OF USE ONLY.

   a. Immunization should be carried out in as cool place as possible, preferably inside a room. If a room is not available, immunization can be carried out in shade and not in direct sun.

b.   Open the carrier **only** when necessary. Remove the vaccine and diluents from the vaccine container, ONLY when necessary.

c.   Take out only one vial of vaccine from the container at a time.

d.   Secure the lid tightly after opening as soon as possible.

e.   Wrap the BCG ampoules in a foil or a dark paper to protect them from heat and light.

f.   Place vials on an ice pack. If no mother or child is waiting put the vials back into the cold chain container until a beneficiary arrives.

g.   When the session is completed, return all vials, open and unopened to the health center.

ix.   In case of Cold Chain Failure

a.   Any vaccine that has NOT been stored at a recommended temperature as per its licensing conditions is no longer a licensed product and should be discarded.

b.   Where there is any doubt that cold chain has not been maintained, vaccines should not be used until further advice has been sought from the vaccine manufacturer.

c.   Vaccine exposed to inappropriate temperatures that is inadvertently administered generally should be repeated.

d.   Vaccine recalls due to inappropriate storage can mean extra doses for patients, increased costs for providers, and damage to public confidence in vaccines.

V. ACCESS CONTROLLED STORAGE

Some products need storage in an access-controlled environment. It is important to identify products that are at risk of theft or abuse or have the potential for addiction, and to provide increased security for those items. This includes products that are in high demand or have the potential for resale (black market value).

Usually, Essential Medicines Lists (EML)/hospital formulary includes several narcotics and psychotropic medicines; one or two will be on facility lists. Typical examples are-

Narcotics: morphine, opium preparations, pethidine, papaverine, hydrocodone and tramadol.

Other opioid and strong analgesics: pentazocine, codeine, dextroproproxyphene and buprenorphine.

Psychotropic drugs: usually the group of drugs called "benzodiazepines," the more common being diazepam, temazepam, nitrazepam, flunitrazepam, and oxazepam. Clonazepam, used to treat epilepsy, may be found under a different class, and is not always under the same control. Strong tranquilizing medicines, such as chlorpromazine, may also be found under this heading.

Note: Other medicines, including antiretroviral used to treat HIV/AIDS, may need storage in a controlled facility, because they are scarce, expensive, and in high demand.

1.   If you have products that need increased security, you must establish access-controlled storage. This will probably include storing the products in-

i.   A separate locked room, cabinet, or safe, or

ii.   A locked wire cage within the storage facility.

2.   Ideally a warning light or bell will be activated if the products are accessed improperly.

3.   Entry to the location of the access-controlled products must be limited to the most senior storekeeper or pharmacist and one other staff member.

4.   Limit the number of keys made for the controlled location and keep a list of people who have keys. For details see Chapter on Handling of Narcotics and Psychotropic Substances.

VI. MEDICAL GASES : SPECIAL CONSIDERATIONS/PRECAUTIONS FOR CYLINDER STORAGE

1. There are two types of hazards associated with medical gas equipment: general fire and explosions, and mechanical issues such as physical damage to compressed gas cylinders.

   Fire and explosions can be caused by incidents involving oxygen, which is the most common gas used in health care facilities, and nitrous oxide, which is used frequently as an inhalation anaesthetic.

   Minimize the use of cylinders, and increase the amount of piped gas used, where necessary.

2. Ensure that all medicinal gases are supplied under compression in metallic cylinder of type confirming to safety regulations.

3. Cylinders should be stored in a special storage room and be kept dry, clean and well ventilated (both top and bottom) and free from materials of flammable nature. Have good access for delivery vehicles and reasonably level floor areas.

4. All equipment supplied for use should be fit for its purpose and must be maintained in a safe and proper manner.

5. Reliable systems should be in place for stock taking and checking of medical gas cylinders, ensuring adequate supplies are always available.

6. Cylinders of medical gases should be stored in accordance with the current guidelines issued by the manufacturers.

7. Requirements for the storage of medical gas cylinders depend on the volume of gas within the cylinders. The greater the volume , the more stringent the requirements for the storage locations. The storage area should be large enough to allow for segregation of full and empty cylinders and permit separation of different medical gases within the store.

8. Storage must be planned so that cylinders can be used in the order in which they are received.

9. Cylinders that are in use must be attached to a cylinder stand or to medical equipment designed to receive and hold cylinders.

10. Cylinders should not be chained to portable or moveable apparatus.

11. Where empty and full cylinders are stored together, empty cylinders must be segregated from full cylinders. Empty cylinders must be marked. This would allow a staff member to be able to quickly identify which cylinders are full and suitable for use when needed in an emergency. Confusion or grabbing an empty cylinder rapidly when one is needed in an emergency could pose a risk to patient safety. Marking empty cylinders is required for the same reason.

12. For cylinders with internal pressure gauges, the facility needs to establish a pressure at which the cylinders will be considered empty.

13. Cylinders stored in the open (outdoors) need to be protected from weather extremes.

14. To keep personnel safe while they work in locations with increased hazards, appropriate `NO SMOKING' signage is required.

15. The supply of medical gases to a patient must be in association with treatment of a medical condition.

16. Minimise risks of confusing oxygen and medical compressed air.

17. Each patient, and appropriate members of the patient's family or care givers, must receive full and proper instruction from a pharmacist or suitably trained person in the safe care and handling of the cylinders and associated equipment.

18. To facilitate recalls of faulty oxygen giving sets, the name, type, serial number and location of each regulator should be recorded and held in the pharmacy.

VII. STORAGE AND HANDLING OF DANGEROUS/ HAZARDOUS MATERIAL

Substance which are ignitable, corrosive, toxic or reactive, are considered hazardous. Proper storage reduces the risk of accidents involving hazardous materials.

A. GENERAL PRINCIPLES OF STORAGE

1. A majority of chemicals and materials fit these categories, acetone, anesthetic ether, alcohols (before dilution), kerosene, antifreeze, insecticides, herbicides, fungicides, cleaning agents, adhesives, arts and craft materials, aerosol cans, propane cylinders, moth repellents, sulphuric acid, laboratory reagents, xylene, potassium permanganate, compressed gases, batteries, etc.

2. Proper segregation is necessary to prevent incompatible materials from inadvertently coming into contact. A physical barrier and/or distance is effective for proper segregation. Store all hazardous materials at separate location under lock and key.

3. Keep minimum quantity of hazardous substances necessary. Purchase only the amount necessary to complete your current job.

4. Large supplies of flammables should never be stored in the same areas as medicines.

5. Store large supplies of flammables in a separate location away from the main storeroom, preferably outside the main storeroom but on the premises and not less than 20 m away from the other buildings. Fire fighting equipment should be easily available.

6. Follow all the storage instructions on the product label. Storage requirements vary based on the hazardous property of the material.

7. Keep all stored chemicals, especially flammable liquids, away from heat and direct sunlight. Flammable liquids each have a flash point, which is the minimum temperature at which the liquid gives off vapor in sufficient concentration to form an ignitable mixture with air near the surface of the liquid. The flash point indicates the susceptibility to ignition.

    i. Acetone and anesthetic ether have a flash point of 18°C.

    ii. Undiluted alcohols have a flash point of 18°C to 23°C. ·

    iii. The flash point for kerosene is 23° to 61°C.

    Note: It is not necessary to store flammable below their flash point, but it is very important to store them in coolest location possible and never in direct sunlight. It is important to control the evaporation rate and avoid the build-up of pressure.

8. Make sure that certain flammable products are stored in the recommended temperature range. The containers will bulge if you store them in temperatures that are too high. Liquid materials will expand, freeze and burst if you store them in temperatures that are too low.

9. Avoid storing chemicals on the floor (even temporarily) or extending into traffic aisles.

10. A small stock of flammables may be kept in a steel cabinet in a well-ventilated area, away from open flames and electrical appliances. Store acids in a dedicated acid cabinet. Nitric acid should be kept isolated from all other acids. Mark the cabinets to indicate that they contain highly flammable liquids, and display the international hazard symbol. In addition, the shelves of the cabinet should be designed to contain and isolate spillage.

11. Do not store chemicals alphabetically except within a grouping of compatible chemicals.

12. Store incompatible substances separately. Corrosive or oxidant substances commonly found in hospitals or other high-level health facilities include trichloroacetic acid, glacial acetic acid, concentrated ammonia solutions, silver nitrate, sodium nitrate, and sodium hydroxide pellets.

13. Always store corrosive substances away from flammables, ideally in a separate steel cabinet to prevent leakage. Use appropriate industrial-type protective gloves and eye-glasses when handling these items.

14. Chemicals should be stored no higher than eye level and never on the top shelf of a storage unit. Do not overcrowd shelves. Each shelf should have an anti-roll lip.

15. Be sure to store all volatile products in well-ventilated areas. Fumes can be toxic to humans and animals.

16. Do not use chemical fume hoods for storage as containers block proper air flow in the hood and reduce available work space.

17. Do periodic maintenance of the storage areas.

B. PREVENTING LEAKAGE OF DANGEROUS MATERIALS/SUBSTANCES

1. Take steps to prevent release or leakage of dangerous substances.

2. Use the original container to store the hazardous material. If the label is lifting off, use a transparent tape to secure it.

3. Liquids should be stored in unbreakable or double-contained packaging, or the storage cabinet should have the capacity to hold the contents if the container breaks.

4. Keep spill kit near to storage areas, and ensuring staff are trained in what to do in the event of a spill.

5. Cleaning up any leaks or spills that occur:

   i. Use a separate broom and dustpan for chemical cleanup. Be sure to lock these tools away when you are not using them.

   ii. Use the right precautions when handling substances - for example, wearing protective clothing or ensuring adequate ventilation.

   iii. Ensure employees who store and handle dangerous substances are properly trained.

   iv. First aid supplies, emergency phone numbers, eyewash and emergency shower equipment, fire extinguishers, spill cleanup supplies and personal protective equipment are readily available.

C. MONITORING OF DANGEROUS MATERIALS

1. Look for problems inside each storage area on a regular basis. Such as:

   i Improper storage of chemicals

   ii. Leaking or deteriorating containers

   iii. Spilled chemicals

   iv. Temperature extremes (too hot or cold in storage area)

    v.   Lack of or low lighting levels

    vi.   Blocked exits or aisles

    vii.   Doors blocked open, lack of security

    viii.   Trash accumulation

    ix.   Open lights or matches

    x.   Fire equipment blocked, broken or missing

    xi.   Lack of information or warning signs ("Flammable liquids", "Acids", "Corrosives", "Poisons", etc.)

2.   Inspect all hazardous material containers. Make sure you can clearly see each label. The containers should be free of rust, bulges, dents or leaks.

VIII. HANDLING OF HAZARDOUS DRUGS (HDs)

1.   Hazardous drugs (HDs) include antineoplastic and cytotoxic agents, immunosuppressants, and antiviral medications. A list of hazardous drugs that require special handling should be posted in every facility providing drug preparation and administration services.

2.   Healthcare workers may be exposed to a hazardous drug at many points–receipt, storage, transportation, preparation, and administration, as well as during waste handling and equipment maintenance and repair. All workers involved in these activities have the potential for contact with hazardous drugs. Routes of unintentional entry of HDs into the body include dermal and mucosal absorption, inhalation, injection, and ingestion (e.g., contaminated foodstuffs, spills, or mouth contact with contaminated hands). Containers of HDs have been shown to be contaminated upon receipt. Both clinical and nonclinical personnel may be exposed to HDs when they handle HDs or touch contaminated surfaces. Table below lists examples of potential routes of exposure based on activity. Workplace exposures to hazardous drugs can cause both acute and chronic health effects, such as skin rashes, adverse reproductive outcomes (including infertility, spontaneous abortions, and congenital malformations), and possibly leukemia and other cancers.

Activities and Potential Opportunity of Exposure to Hazardous Drugs

Receipt	
	• Contacting HD residues present on drug containers, individual dosage units, outer containers, work surfaces, or floors Dispensing. Counting or repackaging tablets and capsules
Compounding and other manipulations	
	• Crushing or splitting tablets or opening capsules
	• Pouring oral or topical liquids from one container to another
	• Weighing or mixing components
	• Constituting or reconstituting powdered or lyophilized HDs
	• Withdrawing or diluting injectable HDs from parenteral containers
	• Expelling air or HDs from syringes
	• Contacting HD residue present on PPE or other garments
	• Deactivating, decontaminating, cleaning, and disinfecting areas contaminated with or suspected to be contaminated with HDs
	• Maintenance activities for potentially contaminated equipment and devices
Administration	
	• Generating aerosols during administration of HDs by various routes (e.g., injection, irrigation, oral, inhalation, or topical application)
	• Performing certain specialized procedures (e.g., intraoperative intraperitoneal injection or bladder instillation)
	• Priming an IV administration set

Patient-care activities
• Handling body fluids (e.g., urine, faeces, sweat, or vomit) or body-fluid-contaminated clothing, dressings, linens, and other materials Spills
• Spill generation, management, and disposal
Transport
• Moving HDs within a healthcare setting
Waste
• Collection and disposal of hazardous waste and trace contaminated waste

3. The health risk depends on the extent of exposure and toxicity of the hazardous drugs. Some epidemiological studies suggest that spontaneous abortions and foetal malformations suffered by nurses who worked in environments in which hazardous drugs were prepared and administered may be related to occupational exposure to these agents. Workers can be protected from exposures to hazardous drugs through engineering and administrative controls, and proper protective equipment.

4. Sources of HDs exposure are leaks, spills, and the creation of aerosols of liquid drugs which can occur during dose preparation.

A. FACILITIES AND ENGINEERING CONTROLS

HDs must be handled under conditions that promote patient safety, worker safety, and environmental protection. Signs designating the hazard must be prominently displayed before the entrance to the HD handling areas.

1. Access to areas where HDs are handled must be restricted to authorized personnel to protect persons not involved in HD handling. HD handling areas must be located away from breakrooms and refreshment areas for personnel, patients, or visitors to reduce risk of exposure.

2. Designated areas must be available for:

    • Receipt and unpacking

    • Storage of HDs

    • Nonsterile HD compounding (if performed by the hospital)

    • Sterile HD compounding (if performed by the hospital) .

3. Certain areas are required to have negative pressure from surrounding areas to contain HDs and minimize risk of exposure. Consideration should be given to uninterrupted power sources (UPS) for the ventilation systems to maintain negative pressure in the event of power loss.

4. Antineoplastic HDs requiring manipulation other than counting or repackaging of final dosage forms and any HD API (active pharmaceutical ingredient) must be stored separately from non-HDs in a manner that prevents contamination and personnel exposure. These HDs must be stored in an externally ventilated, negative-pressure room with at least 12 air changes per hour (ACPH).

5. Non-antineoplastic, reproductive risk only, and final dosage forms of antineoplastic HDs may be stored with other inventory, if permitted by hospital policy.

6. Sterile and nonsterile HDs may be stored together, but HDs used for nonsterile compounding should not be stored in areas designated for sterile compounding to minimize traffic into the sterile compounding area.

7. Engineering controls are required to protect the preparation from cross-contamination and microbial contamination (if preparation is intended to be sterile) during all phases of the compounding process. Engineering controls for containment are divided into three categories representing primary, secondary, and supplementary levels of control. A containment primary engineering control (C-PEC) is a ventilated device designed to minimize worker and environmental HD exposure when directly handling HDs. The containment secondary engineering control (C-SEC) is the room in which the C-PEC is placed. Supplemental engineering controls [e.g., closed-system drug-transfer device (CSTD)] are adjunct controls to offer additional levels of protection.

8. Refrigerated antineoplastic HDs must be stored in a dedicated refrigerator in a negative pressure area with at least 12 ACPH [e.g., storage room, buffer room, or containment segregated compounding area (C-SCA)]. If a refrigerator is placed in a negative pressure buffer room, an exhaust located adjacent to the refrigerator's compressor and behind the refrigerator should be considered.

9. A sink must be available for hand washing. An eyewash station and/or other emergency or safety precautions that meet applicable laws and regulations must be readily available. Water sources and drains must be located at least 1 meter away from the C-PEC.

B. POLICY FOR HANDLING OF HDs

1. Only authorized and adequately trained personnel should receive, prepare, transport, or administer hazardous drugs.

2. A clearly defined orientation and training programme should be completed by every employee who may come into contact with a hazardous drug container. Personnel must be made aware of the unique nature of these agents and the potential risks associated with exposure to them. All employees must be educated regarding the appropriate steps to take in the event of accidental exposure to a hazardous drug. Employees who are pregnant or breastfeeding should be reassigned to areas where contact with these drugs should be avoided.

3. Equipment: Class II vertical flow biohazard cabinets, or biological safety cabinets (BSCs), are currently recommended for preparing hazardous drugs.

4. In addition to the use of BSCs, protective apparel and other supplies designed to minimize the risk of exposure to hazardous drugs must be utilized appropriately. All workers involved in the handling of hazardous drugs should wear powder-free, disposable gloves with reasonable thickness, good fit, and adequate tactile sensation. Some published guidelines recommend double-gloving. Gloves must be changed as soon as possible, if they are contaminated .

5. Labeling, Packaging, Storing, and Transport of HDs from point of Receipt - The safety programme should address the entire lifecycle of HD handling, including receipt, storage, and transportation.

6. Drug packages, bins, shelves, and storage areas for HDs must bear distinctive labels identifying those drugs as requiring special handling precautions.

C. RECEIPT OF HDs

1. All HD APIs (Active Pharmaceutical Ingredient) i.e., the active ingredient contained in medicine, must be unpacked in areas that are neutral/ normal or negative pressure relative to the surrounding areas.

2. HDs must not be removed from their external shipping containers in sterile compounding areas or in any area that is under positive pressure to the surrounding areas.

3. During receipt of HDs, visual examination of cartons for outward signs of damage or breakage is an important initial step in the receiving process.

4. Policies and procedures must be in place for handling damaged cartons or containers of HDs (e.g., returning the damaged goods to the distributor using appropriate containment techniques). These procedures should include the use of PPE. HD spill kits must be available in the receiving area. The spill kit should contain complete PPE, including a respirator, in the event no ventilation protection is available where damaged HD containers are handled. Surgical masks do not provide adequate protection from the harmful effects of these drugs.

5. Damaged shipping containers be transported to a C-PEC designated for nonsterile compounding before opening.

6. Segregation of HD inventory from other drug inventory improves control and reduces the number of staff members potentially exposed to the danger. These HDs must be stored in areas with sufficient external exhaust ventilation (i.e., negative-pressure rooms) having at least 12 air changes per hour.

7. The nonantineoplastic, reproductive risk–only, and HD dosage forms of antineoplastic HDs, may be stored with other inventory if the facility's assessment of risk and policy allow it.

8. HDs placed in inventory should be protected from potential breakage by storage in bins that have high fronts and on shelves that have guards to prevent accidental falling.

9. HDs must be stored to prevent spillage or breakage if the container falls. Special care must also be taken to secure shelves and other storage containers in the event of earthquakes or other natural disasters as appropriate. The bins must also be appropriately sized to properly contain all stock. Care should be taken to separate HD inventory to reduce potential drug errors (e.g., pulling a look-alike vial from an adjacent drug bin).

10. To reduce transfer of HD residue from vials and cartons, all staff members must wear gloves (i.e., chemotherapy gloves).

11. Single chemotherapy gloves are sufficient in receiving, unpacking, and placing HDs into storage, unless there is a spill. Because many studies have shown that HD residue on the drug vial itself is routine and that contamination has been reported in significant amounts, staff should consider wearing double chemotherapy gloves when receiving, unpacking, stocking, and inventorying these drugs and selecting HD packages for further handling.

12. A gown and respiratory protection should also be used when spills or leaks are of concern (e.g., if a carton appears damaged) during HD receiving, unpacking, and storage activities.

D. TRANSPORT OF HDs

1. All transport of HD packages must be done in a manner to reduce environmental contamination in the event of accidental dropping.

2. HD packages must be placed in sealed containers and labeled with a unique identifier. Carts or other transport devices must be designed with guards to protect against falling and breakage.

3. All individuals transporting HDs must have safety training that includes spill control and have spill kits immediately accessible.

4. Staff handling HDs or cleaning areas where HDs are stored or handled must be trained to recognize the unique identifying labels used to distinguish these drugs and areas.

5. Warning labels and signs must be clear to non-English readers. All personnel who work with or around HDs must be trained to appropriately perform their jobs using the established precautions and required PPE.

E. COMPOUNDING AND HANDLING NONSTERILE HD DOSAGE FORMS

1. HDs should be labeled or otherwise identified as such to prevent improper handling.

2. Tablet and capsule forms of HDs should not be placed in automated counting machines, which subject them to stress and may introduce powdered contaminants into the work area.

3. During routine handling of nonsterile HDs and contaminated equipment, workers should wear 2 pairs of gloves.

4. Counting and pouring of HDs should be done carefully, and clean equipment should be dedicated for use with these drugs.

5. Contaminated equipment should be cleaned initially with gauze saturated with sterile water; further cleaned with detergent, sodium hypochlorite solution, and neutralizer; and then rinsed. The gauze and rinse should be contained and disposed of as contaminated waste.

6. Crushing tablets or opening capsules should be avoided; in such cases liquid formulations should be used whenever possible.

7. During the compounding of HDs (e.g., crushing, dissolving, or preparing a solution or an ointment), workers should wear nonpermeable gowns and double gloves. Compounding should take place in a ventilated cabinet.

8. Compounding nonsterile forms of HDs in equipment designated for sterile products must be undertaken with care. Appropriate containment, deactivation, and disinfection techniques must be utilized.

9. HDs should be dispensed in the final dose and form whenever possible. Unit-of-use containers for oral liquids have not been tested for containment properties. Most exhibit some spillage during preparation or use. Caution must be exercised when using these devices.

10. Bulk containers of liquid HDs, as well as specially packaged commercial HDs, must be handled carefully to avoid spills.

F. HD PREPARATION AREA

1. Hazardous drugs should be prepared only in restricted, designated areas. Signs restricting the access of unauthorized personnel are to be prominently displayed. Eating, drinking, smoking, chewing gum, applying cosmetics, and storing food in the preparation area are prohibited.

2. Proper techniques and supplies designed to aid in the safe preparation of hazardous drugs must be utilized at all times.

3. Syringes and IV administration sets with Luer-lock type fittings should be used to prepare and administer hazardous drugs to reduce the potential for accidental leaks or separation of the fittings. Syringes must always be large enough so that they should never be more than three-quarters full. The development of extremes of positive and negative pressure in medication vials must be avoided to reduce the possibility of drug aerosols being introduced into the workspace, e.g. attempting to withdraw 10 ml of fluid from a 10 ml vial or placing 10 ml of a fluid into an air-filled 10 ml vial.

4. Proper aseptic techniques should be followed at all times for worker protection, as well as patient safety. Employees should wash their hands before putting on gloves and again after removing them.

5. A low-permeability, lint-free disposable protective gown with a closed front, long sleeves, and tight-fitting elastic or knit cuffs should be worn at all times when preparing hazardous drugs. This garment should not be worn out of the immediate drug preparation or administration area. Change the gown as soon as possible, if torn or visibly contaminated.

6. If gowns are to be re-used, they must be stored in a manner that does not permit potential contact between outer and inner surfaces.

7. Dispose off all used gowns, gloves and disposable materials used in preparation by placing them in red bags.

G. HD ADMINISTRATION

1. Only individuals trained in the administration of HDs should do so. Nurses who administer HDs and care for patients receiving chemotherapy should meet the requirements of the Oncology Nursing. During administration, access to the administration area should be limited to patients receiving therapy and essential personnel.

2. Eating, drinking, applying makeup, and the presence of foodstuffs should be avoided in patient care areas while HDs are administered.

3. For inpatient therapy, where lengthy administration techniques may be required, hanging or removing HDs should be scheduled to reduce exposure of family members and ancillary staff and to avoid the potential contamination of dietary trays and personnel. Because much of the compounding and administration of HDs are done in outpatient or clinic settings with patients and their family members near the compounding area, care must be taken to minimize environmental contamination and to maximize the effectiveness of cleaning (decontamination) activities.

4. The design of such areas must include surfaces that are readily cleaned and decontaminated. Upholstered and carpeted surfaces should be avoided, as they are not readily cleaned. Several studies have shown floor contamination and the ineffectiveness of cleaning practices on both floors and surfaces.

5. HDs may also be administered in nontraditional locations, such as the operating room, which presents challenges in training of personnel and in proper containment of the drugs and drug residue. Intracavitary administration of HDs (e.g., into the bladder, peritoneal cavity, or chest cavity) frequently requires equipment for which locking connections may not be available. Inhalation of some HDs to treat certain diseases also has the potential for significant worker exposure as well as environmental contamination, as closed system administration is problematic.

H. HD SPILL MANAGEMENT

1. All staff members who handle HDs should receive safety training that includes recognition of HDs and appropriate spill response. HD spill kits, containment bags, and disposal containers must be available in all areas where HDs are handled. Supplies for emergency treatment (e.g., soap, eyewash, sterile saline for irrigation) should be immediately located in any area where HDs are stored, compounded, or administered.

2. Equipment Needed: Chemotherapy/hazardous drug spill kit (should be available in Pharmacy Store Room), including:

   a. Tyvek gown or coveralls

   b. Shoe covers

    c.   Splash goggles

    d.   Two pairs of chemotherapy tested disposable gloves

    e.   Absorbent pads

    f.   Scoop with detachable scraper for collecting glass fragments

    g.   Two 5 gallon plastic waste disposal bags

    h.   One Ziploc bag for returning contaminated splash goggles to Pharmacy

    i.   Hazardous Drug Waste labels

3.   Alert nearby persons about the spill. Pregnant employees should leave the area during clean up.

4.   If HD spill splashes on skin, eyes, or clothing:

    i.   Call for help, if needed.

    ii.   Immediately remove contaminated clothing and prevent risk of additional skin contact with the spilled drug.

    iii.   Flood affected eye with water or isotonic eyewash for at least 15 minutes.

    iv.   Inform the appropriate area manager.

    v.   Clean affected skin with soap (not a disinfectant cleanser) and water; rinse thoroughly.

    vi.   Obtain medical attention.

5.   Obtain chemotherapy/hazardous drugs spill kit.

6.   Put on safety goggles and double gloves from kit. If spill involves more than 5 mL or covers more than one square foot (or, for smaller spills, at the discretion of the person cleaning the spill), put on Tyvek gown and shoe covers (or coveralls) from kit. Tuck sleeves into the outer gloves.

7.   If there are broken glass fragments, use the detachable scraper to carefully "sweep" them or other sharps into the scoop. Place glass fragments in the puncture-resistant HD waste container.

8.   Use the absorbent pads to gently cover and wipe up the spilled material. Spill cleanup should proceed progressively from areas of lesser to greater contamination. Completely remove and place all contaminated material in the disposal bags.

9.   Rinse the area with water and then clean with detergent, sodium hypochlorite solution, and neutralizer or other validated decontamination solution. Rinse the area three times (Housekeeping can be called in for this step ONLY) and place all materials used for containment and cleanup in disposal bags. Seal bags and place them in the appropriate final container for disposal as hazardous waste

10.   Place any contaminated hospital linens in a hospital laundry bag.

11.   Place other (personal) contaminated clothing in a sealed plastic bag. If it will be laundered, double bag for transport, then wash twice before combining with other laundry. If it will be discarded, place it in the open bag from the spill kit.

12.   Remove the shoe covers (if used) and outer pair of gloves. Place these into the open bag from the spill kit.

13.   Remove the goggles and place them into the open bag from the spill kit. (Alternately, goggles may be washed and reused.)

14.   Close the open waste bag (by knotting or using twist tie or tape), then place it into the second clear 5-gallon bag from the spill kit.

15. Remove the Tyvek gown (or coveralls) and inner gloves. Place these into the second bag from the spill kit. Close the outer bag.

16. Wash hands thoroughly.

17. Disposal instructions for spills of chemotherapeutic or regulated hazardous drugs to be followed.

18. Document exposure in employee's medical record and medical surveillance log.

19. Report ALL incidents.

10 | Inventory Management

An inventory is a list of all the items, goods, materials and equipment that are kept at the health facility. The person in charge of the health facility should keep a master copy of all items and update this list each time an item is received and issued.

An effective inventory management system apart from keeping track of receipts and issues for discharge of an accounting responsibility, acts as an instrument in improving health care and is a pre-requisite for optimal stock management. Key issues in inventory management are service level and safety level. A judicious balance has to be struck between these two to ensure that while on the one hand funds do not get locked up in inventory holding, on the other, no stock-outs occur. Apart from the carrying cost, wastage due to excessive orders and time expiring stocks add to the overall cost of medicines in a meagre resource setting where aim is to optimize resources for ensuring maximum reach of the finances. A proper scientific management of inventory thus assumes paramount importance. Accurate stock records is a pre-requisite for effective inventory management.

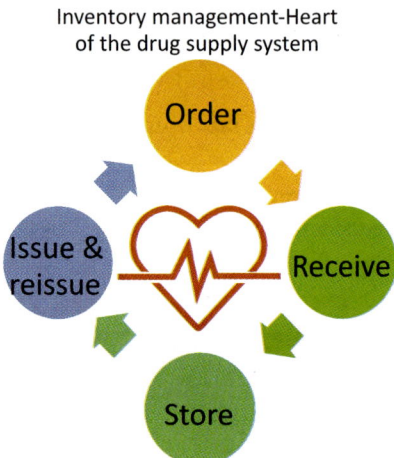

Inventory management-Heart of the drug supply system

Accurate stock records is a pre-requisite

Factors contributing to inaccurate stock records

High volume, repetitious entries

Loans not documented

Drugs names and descriptions are similar

Duplicate entries for receipts or issues/forgotten indents

Spoiled or junk stock destroyed but not written off

Theft produces inaccurate records, except when deliberately altered to conceal the theft

Physical count rarely or never taken, or records not reconciled after stock count

Sloppy warehouse conditions

Minimal supervision of warehouse staff

I. STANDARD LIST OF STOCK ITEMS

1. Each medical store should maintain a standard list of stock items that includes all products

they handle, with their specifications, including form, strength, and quantity per package. The list should be regularly updated and distributed to sub-stores and units.

2. Do not order products that are not on the standard list unless you have special permission. Do not accept deliveries of products not on the list unless special circumstances have been identified.

3. Inventory records should be maintained for all products on the list.

4. Double accounting systems should be followed: both bin cards in the stores, and parallel ledgers outside.

5. Essentially bin cards and ledgers should be maintained by two different persons.

6. As per established practice, bin cards should be posted simultaneously as and when any transaction takes place. For big hospitals with multiple indenting sources, this requirement can be dispensed with.

7. Discrepancies in the records to be reconciled with the full knowledge of the Medical Officer/Officer in-charge Stores.

II. STOCK RECORDS

Stock records: A generic term that applies to bin cards, Kardex records, stock ledgers, and computer files. These provide basic information for inventory management providing all transactions for an item, including receipts, issues, orders placed, orders received, and stock losses. Many supply system maintain two stock records for each item, to improve accuracy and accountability. Typically, there is a bin card kept with the stock, combined with a ledger, kardex, or computer system kept in the central office.

In most supply systems, computerization is desirable if the local situation can support automation. Computer are essential to manage an inventory of any size with perpetual purchasing. Moreover, a good software programme properly used makes information retrieval and reports much easier than a manual system. However, stock can still be controlled with manual records in most drug supply environments, if necessary.

The key point about stock records, whether manual or computerized, is that they must be current and accurate. It is impossible to manage the reordering process well, if stock movement cannot be tracked.

1. The minimal information that should be collected on stock records (manual or computerized) for medicines and other health products includes:

   i. Product name/description (including the form [e.g. capsule, tablet, liquid suspension, etc.] and strength)

   ii. Stock on hand/beginning stock balance

   iii. Receipts

   iv. Issues

   v. Losses/adjustments

   vi. Closing/ending balance

   vii. Transaction reference (e.g. issue voucher number or name of supplier or recipients).

2. Depending on the system, stock records might also include additional product information such as-

   i. Special storage conditions (e.g., 2°-8°C)

   ii. Unit prices

   iii. Lot numbers/bin locations

   iv. Item codes

   v. Expiry dates

3. A logistics information system must have three different types of records: stock-keeping records, transaction records, and consumptions records. See Appendix 3-5 for sample forms of each. Clinic-level facilities may use other forms in addition to these.

4. Stock records might also include certain calculated data items. These are determined by mathematical formulas, that depend on system design parameters (e.g., how often orders are placed). Calculated data items include-

   i. Consumption data, such as average monthly consumption (C_A)

   ii. Lead times for ordering/requisition

   iii. Maximum and minimum stock levels

   iv. Reorder quantities and reorder interval

   v. Emergency order point.

5. A storage and distribution system may not necessarily use all these forms, but it will need forms to record stock-keeping data and product transactions. Standard forms used for inventory control include-

   i. Stock cards

   ii. Bin cards with each product as duplicate record and should be kept physically with the stock

   iii. Requisition/issue vouchers

   iv. Receiving forms (packing slip/freight bill)

   v. Delivery /issue vouchers

   vi. Expired stock disposal forms

   vii. Physical inventory forms

   viii. List of approved medicines and prices.

III. SELECTIVE INVENTORY CONTROL METHODS

1. Selective inventory control is an essential part of the material management. It is difficult to apply uniform control over all items. as hundreds or thousands of individual transactions are carried out each year. To do their job effectively, materials manager must avoid the distraction of unimportant details and concentrate on significant matters. Therefore, selective control emphasizes on the variations in methods of control from item to item based on selective basis such as cost, criticality, availability, difficulty in procurement, consumption, etc. Thus, allowing focusing effort more on items that are key to the organization, and applying lesser control on other items.

2. Several classification systems are used for selective treatment of various types of materials (see below). According to the nature of the inventories carried by an organization, a suitable method of classification should be chosen.

Inventory control methods

	Basis	Main uses
ABC Always better control	Value of consumption	To control inventory
VED Vital Essential Desirable	Critically of the drug	To determine the stocking levels
XYZ	Value of items in storage	To review inventory & uses at scheduled intervals
HML High Medium Low	Unit cost of the material	To control purchases
FSN Fast, Slow, Not moving	Consumption pattern	To control obsolescence
SDE Scarce Difficult Easy	Problems faced in procurement	Lead-time analysis and purchasing strategies
SOS Season Off season	Nature of supplies	Procurement/holding strategies
GOLF Govt Ordinary Local Foreign	Source of material	Procurement strategies

3. For details of ABC analysis and VED principles. For details see Chapter on Quantification of medical supplies.

	All these funds spent on	Items
Class A Items - Highest Unit Cost/ Highest Volume Items; Account for 75% of value of drugs purchased	Highest potential for saving	Comprise 20% of the total items
Class B Items (Consume 15%) Moderate value inventory items	Some additional savings possible	Comprise 50% of the total items
Class C Items (Low Cost/Low Volume Items); Account for 10% of value of drugs purchased	High management inputs required for no cost reduction	Comprise 100% of the total items

4. Combination approach or hybrid methods use combination of the two categories like a matrix combining ABC and VED categories or HML and VED categories or XYZ and FSN categories or ABC and XYZ categories (see below). ABC and VED matrix is more relevant in hospitals. The AV category becomes the most important for inventory control because the items are very much cost consuming being a category and also vital for uses. These items can be controlled

by the top-level management. The CD category items are not very costly and at the same time of desirable category. These items are controlled at the lower level.

ABC-VED matrix

Class	V items	E items	D items
A items	Constant control Regular follow-up Forecast carefully	Moderate stocks	Nil stocks Min Service level
B Items	Moderate stocks	Moderate stocks	Very low stocks
C items	High stocks Max Service level	Moderate stocks	Low stocks

HML-VED Matrix

Class	V items	E items	D items
H	Defibrillator	X-ray machine	Air- curtains
M	Ventilator	Electric cautery	Ultrasonic wash machine
L	Oxygen regulator	Patient trolley	Electronic BP machine

XYZ-FSN matrix

Class	F items	S items	D items
X items	Tight inventory control	Reduce stock to very los levels	Quick disposal of items at good price
Y items	Normal inventory control	Low levels of control	Dispose off as early as possible
Z items	Reduce clerical labour by increasing stocks	Low levels of stocks	Dispose off at lower cost as well

IV. SERVICE LEVEL AND SAFETY STOCK REQUIREMENTS

1. Reducing the safety stock increases the chance of stock-outs. Therefore, the cost of additional safety stock must be weighed against the potential health impact of stock-outs.

2. The effect of safety stock can be measured in terms of the service level. This is defined as the percentage of requests that can be filled from stock-in hand. For example, a 95% service level means that a specific drug is in stock 95% of the time on average. The companion to this concept is the stock-out frequency—A 95% service corresponds with a stock-out frequency of 5%.

3. The service level in its most representative form is the percentage of individual items ordered from supplier or warehouse that is issued form stock on hand. This is measured by counting the total number of items issued and divided by the total number of items requested.

   Service level = (# items issued /# items requested) × 100

4. This level of safety stock required to assure a given service level is based on mathematical probabilities and is demonstrate in Figure below. The point to note is that the cost of safety stock required increases very steeply with the highest service levels.

5. There are many ways of estimating the safety stock required to achieve specific service levels. The more precise methods require historical date on consumption patterns, (which may not be always available).

6. The simplest approach is to establish arbitrary levels and then to adjust them on the basis of delivery lead times, an experience with different types of drugs, particularly knowledge of seasonal demand and of the VED category of the product (Vital, Essential or Desirable). Obviously the longer the lead time, or the more vital the drug, the greater the safety stock needs to be. A reasonable starting point might be as shown in table as below.

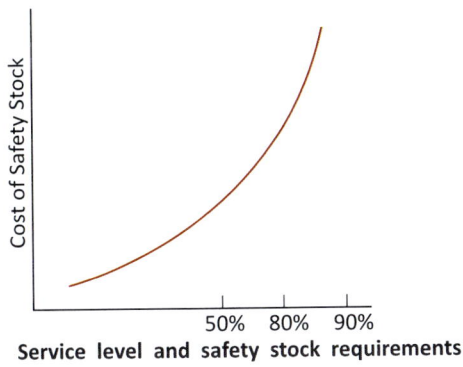

Safety Stock Requirements in relation to Lead Time

Lead Time	Safety Stock
1 month	2 weeks' usage
2 months	4 weeks' usage
3 months	5 weeks' usage
4 months	6 weeks' usage
6 months	8 weeks' usage
8 months	9 weeks' usage
12 months	12 weeks'

7. Carefully kept inventory records should indicate stock levels, and the frequency and duration of stock-outs. These records can be used to adjust safety stocks upward or downward. For the purpose of sizing pharmaceutical warehouses it is best to over-estimate safety stocks. The aim is to ensure that adequate space is available should safety stock levels to be revised upwards.

V. PHYSICAL INVENTORY

A physical inventory is the process of counting by hand the number of each type of product in the store at any given time. A physical inventory helps ensure that the stock balances recorded on stock-keeping records match the quantities of products actually in the store.

There are two kinds of physical inventory:

Cyclic inventory

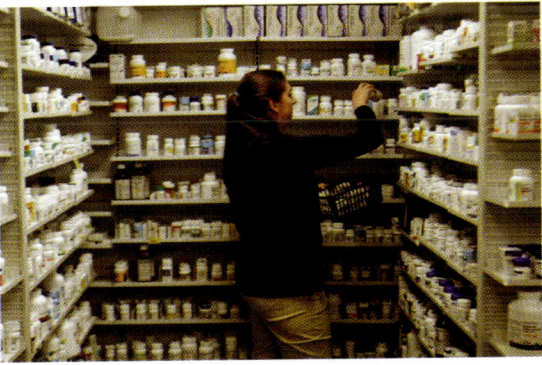

Complete physical inventory: All products are counted at the same time. A complete inventory should be taken at least once a year. More frequent inventory (quarterly or monthly) is recommended for large warehouses, this may require closing the storage facility for a day or longer.

Cyclic or random physical inventory: Selected products are counted and checked against the stock-keeping records on a rotating or regular basis throughout the year. This process is also called cycle counting. The best approach to tracking the quantity actually in stock is cyclic counting and is superior to annual counting.

A complete physical inventory is easier to conduct regularly at facilities that manage smaller quantities of products. Cyclic or random physical inventory is usually appropriate at facilities that manage larger quantities of products.

When conducting a physical inventory, count each product individually by generic name, dosage form, and strength.

1. **Cyclic physical inventory (continuous counting) can be organized in many ways:**
   i. **Dosage form:** Count tablets in January, capsules in February, liquids in March, etc.
   ii. **Location in the storeroom:** Count shelves 1-4 in January, 5-8 in February, etc.
   iii. **Time availability:** Count a few items each day whenever staff has time.
   iv. **ABC category wise counting:** A items three or four times a year, B items twice, and C items once; it may be worth adding to the A category any B or C items that are prone to disappear.
   v. **Stock on hand:** On a periodic basis, count each item for which stock on hand is at or below the minimum inventory level. This method may be faster, since there are smaller quantities to count.

2. If cyclic physical inventory is used, count each product at least once during the year. Count fast-moving items and full supply products more frequently.

3. **Steps in conducting a physical inventory:**
   i. **Plan.**
      a. For a complete physical inventory, schedule the day(s) and time.
      b. For a cyclic or random physical inventory, identify which products will be counted and the corresponding time period for those products.
   ii. **Assign staff.**
   iii. **Organize the storeroom.**
      a. Arrange products according to FEFO.
      b. Make sure open cartons and boxes are visible.
      c. Separate damaged or expired products.
   iv. **Count the usable products.**
      a. Count products according to the units by which they are issued (e.g., tablet or pieces) not by the carton or box.
      b. Estimate quantities in open containers for products packaged in bulk. If a bottle of 1,000 capsules is 2/3 full, estimate 650 or 700 capsules. If you have a one liter bottle of syrup that is ½ full, estimate 0.5 L.
   v. For best results, the staff who is counting should not be the ones to reconcile discrepancies. A system of rotating different staff through both functions help maintain the integrity of the process.

4. **Update the stock-keeping records.**
   a. Write the date of the physical inventory and the words "Physical Inventory."
   b. Using a different colour ink, write the quantity of the product that you counted during stock-taking.

5. **Take action based on the results of the physical inventory.**
   i. If the results of the physical inventory differ from the balance on the stock/bin card, update the balance by adding or subtracting the excess or missing quantities.
   ii. Dispose of damaged or expired products found during the physical inventory according to procedures laid down.
   iii. For either of the above, identify, document, and correct the cause of the problem.

6. **Discuss the findings of the inventory with the facility staff.**
   - Congratulate the staff, if appropriate.
   - Take corrective actions, if required.

VI. STOCK ROTATION AND CONTROL

When issuing products, it is important to follow the First Expiry First Out (FEFO) policy. Remember, the order in which products are received is not necessarily the order in which they will expire. Products you received most recently may expire sooner than the products you received earlier. So, it is extremely important to always check the expiry dates and to make sure the dates are visible while the products are in storage. Following FEFO minimizes wastage from product expiry.

1. Always issue products that will expire first, ensuring they are not too close to or past their expiration date. The shelf life remaining must be sufficient for the product to be used before the expiry date.

2. To have access to drugs with shorter expiry date first, put these in front shelves. Those with longer expiry date should be placed behind those with shorter dates.

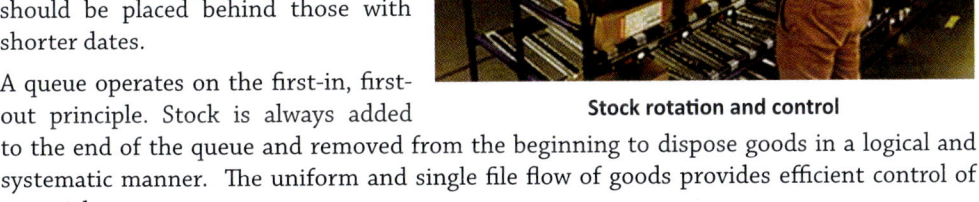

Stock rotation and control

3. A queue operates on the first-in, first-out principle. Stock is always added to the end of the queue and removed from the beginning to dispose goods in a logical and systematic manner. The uniform and single file flow of goods provides efficient control of materials.

4. Issue materials without an expiry date using first-in, first out (FIFO) principle and mark these with the date of receipt.

5. The pharmacist must check medicines for expiry while indenting from the stores.

6. Store-in-charge should maintain a register for expiry dates of drugs and write expiry dates on stock cards. If stock management software is being used, drugs nearing expiry report should be generated every month.

7. Inspection and store checks – The specialists/medical officer in-charge and the dispensing pharmacists must check the register on drug expiry and substantiate physically every month so that there is no discrepancy between the register and physical stock and duly certify in the drug expiry register.

8. Provide details of the items with quantity in stock and date of expiry to the specialists/medical officers to enable consumption of such drugs at least 3–6 months before the due date of expiry. Update this list every month and should be duly acknowledged every month by the Specialist/Medical Officer in-charge concerned.

9. Ensure that out-of –date stock procedure is followed by clearly marking them in black and segregate them from in-date stock, until rearrangement can be made to have the out-of-date stock destroyed.

10. Take non-usable and expired medications off the shelf and store in a separate, secure area under the control of pharmacy, until final disposal. For details of disposal method see section on Handling of Expired Medicines.

Internal transfer/inter-inventory mechanism

1. It is important that drugs are not allowed to expire in the health facility because of changes in disease pattern or for any other reasons.

2. Items that can be used elsewhere should be transferred immediately from one health facility to another for subsequent redistribution through proper indents.

3. Excess stock should be transferred at least 1–3 months before expiry of the item.

4. Detailed list of drugs due to expire, with quantity available should be shared with other hospitals/health centers in respective districts and the office of the CMO concerned, through mail for effective timely circulation.

VII. ORDERLY ARRANGEMENT OF MEDICINES

1. Medical stores must have a system for classifying or organizing medicines, and must ensure that all employees know the system being used.

   ### a. Fixed Location

   In a fixed location system, each stock item is allocated to specific shelves, pallet racking, or an area of floor. A fixed location system is like a house in which each family member has his or her own room. A room is left empty if the person is not at home. With a fixed location system, stock administration is relatively easy. Goods can always be found in the same place. Disadvantages of this system are inflexibility and if there is a change in the quantity ordered or a change in packaging, assigned location may become too large or too small, with lack of space for new item or waste of space because at times it is largely empty.

   ### b. Fluid Location

   In a fluid system, the store is divided into many designated locations. Each location is assigned a code. Individual items are stored wherever space is available at the time of delivery. A fluid location system is like a hotel. Rooms are assigned only when guests arrive.

   A fluid location system uses available space efficiently, but it requires sophisticated stock administration. Experience suggests that a store using a fluid location system can be 20 to 25% smaller than one using a fixed location system. Stock administration requires following:

   - The procurement unit provides information on the type, volume, and weight of goods arriving
   - The storekeeper assesses which locations will be empty when the new stock arrives and assigns a suitable location. These data are recorded in the stock control system.
   - If insufficient space is available, other goods may be moved to more space.
   - The stock control location records are updated.

   ### c. Semi-fluid Location

   A semi-fluid location system is a combination of the previous two. It is a hotel that has regular guests. Regular guests are always given the same room. Casual guests are given any room that is available. In a semi-fluid system, each item is assigned some fixed space for picking stock. When an order is prepared, the order-picking staffs know where to find each item. The remainder of the store is filled on the fluid location principle. When the picking stock runs low, the fixed locations are restocked from the fluid locations.

2. Within the area for each form, a fixed, fluid, or semi-fluid system is used for arranging items in the store. Some common system for arranging medicines include-

   i. **Alphabetical order by generic name:** Often seen in both large and small facilities. When using this system, the labeling must be changed when the EML/Hospital formulary is revised or updated.

   ii. **Therapeutic or pharmacologic category:** Most useful in small storerooms or dispensaries where the storekeeper is very knowledgeable about pharmacology.

   iii. **Dosage form:** Medicines come in different forms, such as tablets, syrups, injectables, and external use products such as ointments and creams. In this system, medicines are categorized according to their dosage form.

Arrangement of stocks

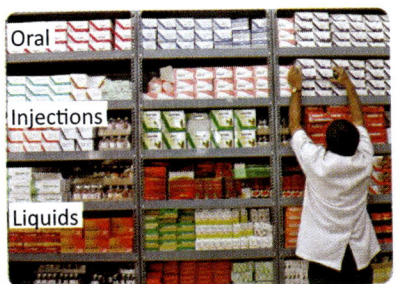
By dosage forms

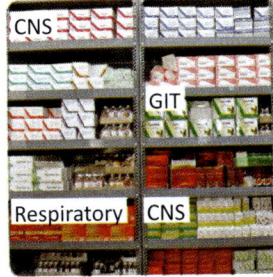
By therapeutic class

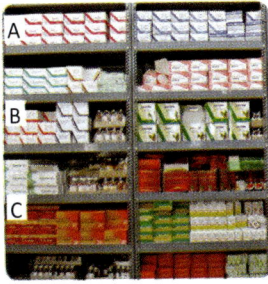
In alphabetical order: by generic or brand names

   iv. **Level of use:** Items for different levels of the health care system are kept together. This works well in stores at a higher level when storage of kits is required.

   v. **Frequency of use:** Frequently used products that move quickly or often through the store should be placed in the front of the room or closest to the staging area. This system should be used in combination with another system.

   vi. **Random bin:** Identifies a specific storage space or cell with a code that corresponds to its aisle, shelf, and position on the shelf. For example, a shelving unit can be divided into cells, each with a unique location code. A unit of shelving might be labeled "A", its bays "A1" and "A2" and its shelves "A", "B" and "C" A unique cell would be identified as A1-A, A2-B. This cell is called a bin. This method is a combination of the methods described above; stored items are placed alphabetically within therapeutic classification by generic name; if there are more than one brand name of the same generic drug, all are stored in the bin for that type. This system requires computer automation.

   vii. **Item coding:** Each item has its own article and location code. This system has the greatest flexibility, but it is also the most abstract. Stores staff do not need any technical knowledge of the products to manage this system because the codes contain the information needed for storing product properly, such as temperature requirements, level of security, and flammability. This system works well in computerized inventory control systems.

3. Periodic stock counts should be performed to check, if medicines have expired.

4. Products approaching their expiry dates must be removed from usable stock and neither be dispensed nor supplied. All stock which has expired and cannot be returned to the

manufacturer, must be destroyed following guidelines (see section on expired drug & waste disposal):

    i.   To prevent accidental usage or such medicine coming into the possession of unauthorized persons,

    ii. In such a manner as not to cause harm or potential harm to the environment.

5.   Sterile products with broken seals and/or damaged packaging, and stock suspected of possible contamination, must neither be dispensed nor supplied.

6.   Stock which is contaminated or withheld from supply and which is not destroyed immediately must be kept separately from usable stock so that it cannot be dispensed in error and that leakage from damaged packaging cannot contaminate other medicines.

7.   The quality system should ensure that the right products are delivered to the right addressee within a satisfactory time period.

8.   A tracing system must enable any faulty product to be found and an effective recall procedure must be in place.

9.   These procedures should be approved, signed and dated by the person responsible for the quality system, the logistics manager and the responsible pharmacist.

VIII. ACTIVITY REPORTS AND PERFORMANCE MONITORING

The most accurate stock records have little value it the information in them is not compiled in reports for use by the managers who make purchasing and stock management decisions. Routine reports on purchasing and inventory management activities should be produced monthly to quarterly in a computerized system and at least annually in manual system. The following lists illustrate the types of reports that are useful for improving inventory management:

1.   Storage facilities should report on

    i.   Stock position - stock on hand and on order, globally and by item, reported as absolute quantities and in items of months' worth of consumption.

    ii. Beginning and ending inventory value, and the average inventory holding costs.

    iii. Changes in inventory value and any discrepancies noted during stock counts.

    iv. Consumption patterns for all stock items and an ABC analysis of consumption with computer assistance, this can be done globally and for each operating unit.

    v.   Service level from suppliers to medical stores and from medical stores to health facilities.

    vi. Expiry status of drugs in inventory and estimate of how much stock is likely to expire before it can be used.

    vii. Quantity and value of obsolete stock waiting for disposal and stock destroyed or junked.

IX. MANAGEMENT INFORMATION SYSTEM (MIS) IN DRUG MANAGEMENT

Computers have revolutionalized many aspects of drug management. Computers can be used in all aspects of the drug management cycle, from selection to use. They are capable of generating forms, reports, tables, graphs, and charts. Using communication devices, users can exchange or share this information with other computers at the same site via local area network (LAN) or with computers anywhere in the world.

When used effectively, computer systems save money, promote efficiency, and improve the quality of services. However, poorly conceived or implemented computer systems waste money, decrease efficiency, and distract attention from other management improvements.

A. BENEFITS AND LIMITATIONS OF MIS

1. Some of the benefits of computerization & MIS are to:

    i. Simplify and speed up complex tasks

    ii. Increase accuracy by checking spelling, calculations, and data integrity

    iii. Update and access information quickly

    iv. Automate repetitive tasks

    v. Provide management information for decision making

    vi. Allow organizations to expand the volume and scope of operations

    vii. Streamline administrative processes

    viii. Generate timely reports without repeated efforts in compiling data.

2. Limitations of computers & MIS are that they cannot assume responsibilities, make decisions, define problems, set objectives, improve the basic data available, or make a person more organized. They cannot fulfill needs, if appropriate hardware and software are not chosen, and they are not a one-time expense: funds are required for upgrades, training, and support over time for both hardware and software.

B. KEY STEPS IN THE COMPUTERIZATION PROCESS

1. Identify the tasks or the system to be computerized with a detailed analysis of needs versus current systems.

2. Survey the environment and consider integrating with other systems to the extent feasible (what software and hardware are being used by other departments? Is there an institutional computer policy? What equipment is already available?)

3. Evaluate the staff situation (actual versus needed).

4. Select software before hardware.

5. Language of the software is appropriate. Identify whether the software needed is available in the local language and to which original version it is equivalent (non-English-language versions are sometimes not as current as English versions).

6. Ensure the availability of supplies and maintenance.

7. Select the hardware and software suppliers that provide the most support.

8. Plan progressive implementation (one step at a time) and involve current and future users in the design and implementation process.

C. FEATURES OF PROCUREMENT AND INVENTORY MANAGEMENT SOFTWARE

1. **General features of Procurement and Inventory Software**

    Security: restricts user: access to a particular module with password protection

    Allows multiple users

    Uses various pricing options

    Automates backup routines

    Checks data integrity (for example, it is impossible to enter a letter or other character, if a number is expected, and vice versa)

    Links with a full accounting package

    Exports data such as to spreadsheet for specific analysis

    Data retention plan

2. **Specific: Features of Procurement Software**

   Manages simultaneous tenders

   Generates all tender documents

   Manages bids and purchase orders in multiple currencies

   Compares bids using a common unit regardless of pack size variation

   Generates contracts and purchases orders for suppliers

   Monitors order status and payments

   Monitors supplier performance (lead time; contract price versus invoiced price)

   Generates receiving reports

   Updates inventory databases

3. **Specific Features of Inventory Software**

   Tracks monthly consumption

   Keeps track of stock out periods

   Calculates average monthly consumption, taking into consideration past consumption and stock out periods

   Calculates minimum and maximum stock levels

   Calculates optimum reorder level, taking into consideration minimum stock, actual stock balance, lead time, procurement and forecasting periods and outstanding orders, as well as user-defined maximum and minimum stock levels

   Monitors expiry dates by lot

   Generates lists by location

   Manages distribution according to expiry due and/or location

   Monitors clients' consumption and budget

   Allows multiple purchase and selling prices, as well as the possibility to enter discounts, surcharges and taxes

   Generates audit report

   Generates ABC analysis report

D. THE OUTPATIENT PHARMACY MANAGEMENT SOFTWARE

The Pharmacy Management system (PMS) otherwise referred to as the pharmacy information system stores data, systemizes and controls the use of the medication process with the pharmacies. The prime purpose of a PMS is to assist the pharmacist in the safe and effective delivery of pharmaceutical drugs.

These systems may be an independent software for the pharmacy's use only, or in a hospital setting, pharmacies may be integrated within an inpatient hospital computer physician order entry (CPOE) system. To perform core duties effectively the pharmacy requires some core features in the software:

1. **Report:** The reports offer valuable insights into the operations in the pharmacy as pharmacies interact with multiple patients every day, and data regarding each of these interactions are stored within the pharmacy information system which may be needed during a certification or inspection process.

   It can be used to distinguish the patients who visit the pharmacy frequently for refills, fast moving items and this can be used to stock accordingly.

2. **Dispensing work flow management:** The pharmacist can also perform pre-checks by reviewing prescription for potential drug interactions, appropriate dosage, duplicate therapies, or transcription errors.

3. **E-prescription & Pre-checks:** E-prescriptions provide a user-friendly option for the patients by dispensing the right medicine and thus reducing the risk of errors due to illegible handwritten prescriptions. The electronic prescription feature can be used by the pharmacy to manage refills and allows doctors to send the new refills directly into the pharmacy management system, allowing rapid dispensing of the medicines.

4. **SMS and Notification:** With the use of a pharmacy management system, the pharmacist can schedule text messages to be sent to patients intimating them before their prescriptions running out. The patients can then let the pharmacist if they need a refill, simply by responding to the message. The status updates allows the pharmacist to keep in touch with the patients, ensuring patient satisfaction.

5. **Multi-Store and Multi-Location Support:** Stores at multiple locations can easily be managed with a pharmacy information system as data about stock levels, sales, returns from multiple stores can be viewed in a single software. Overall reports for the entire chain of stores can be generated, giving the user a complete overview of profit, loss, stock levels, etc.

6. **User Management Module:**

   Access to various features can be limited for different users, for easy management allowing for restricted access to various users. This authentication is classified into two conditions namely:

   Administrator User: The user can control the buying and selling process, list the medicines, view the stock and perform other tasks. The user is able to view the pharmacy list and plays an essential role in controlling the sales and stocks being processed every day.

   Administrator Authentication User: The users who are authenticated can view all processes including selling reports, transactions, modification of the medicine list and the medicine stock. This feature also helps to track regular activities and generate daily accounts by utilizing the multi-site software.

Tips for stock storage and record keeping

- Assign responsibility for stock control and the store room and develop written procedures.
- Keep the store room tidy and well organised. An organised store saves time when ordering or locating items and prevents stock from getting lost.
- Avoid wastage by rotating stock according to expiry dates and FIFO.
- Store drugs, medical supplies and equipment separately, if possible in a different store room, from linen, food and non-medical supplies.
- Make sure store records are completed regularly.
- Keep stock cards in the storeroom. This enables the person responsible for stock control to update the cards after every transaction (ordering, receiving and issuing stock). Write each transaction on a separate line, even if there is more than one transaction on the same day.
- Record any stock-outs on stock cards and report these to your supervisor.
- Store stock cards together in a box or keep each card with the stock in the correct place on the shelves.
- Keep and file old cards.
- Carry out random checks to ensure that record cards are being updated regularly and accurately.
- Generate reports from time-to-time to take stock of situation and review such as stock position, inventory value, consumption pattern, expiry status, etc.

11 | Handling of Narcotics and Psychotropic Drugs

Specific legislation exists in relation to Schedule X drugs such as morphine, ketamine, barbiturates, etc. These are substances or products as specified in Schedule X of Drugs and Cosmetics Act, that are subject to control under several legislations to prevent their misuse by obtaining illegally or causing addiction. Narcotics and Psychotropic Substances (NDPS) Act as amended is concerned with control and regulation of operations relating to Narcotic Drugs and Psychotropic Substances. The Amended NDPS Act 2014 expanded the scope of the Act to include medical and scientific use and prepared a notified list of Essential Narcotic Drug [ENDs] for medical and scientific use and transferred the power to regulate ENDs to Central Controller. ENDs approved by the Drug Controller General of India includes morphine, Methadone, Codeine, Hydrocodone, Oxycodone, and Fentanyl. It defined the criteria for Recognized Medical Institutions (RMI) with criteria for stocking and dispensing opioids for medical use and conferred the power of recognition of medical institution (RMIs) to State Drugs Controller. This authorization of RMIs is for a period of 3 years and renewable from the same agency. For ENDs a designated medical practitioner in-charge is appointed/designated to ensure stocks, security, record, reports; estimation of requirement – and amendments from time-to-time. One should be aware of this legislation and comply with the Governments' policy regarding the ordering, collection, storage and administration of ENDs. RMIs should submit the annual return (Form 3I) before 31st of March of every year even if they have not used any ENDs in the preceding year.

A. GUIDELINES FOR DEALING WITH ESSENTIAL NARCOTIC DRUGS (ENDs)

Distribution of ENDs should be undertaken from licensed premises. In order to handle and dispense ENDs, the personnel should also be licensed by the Ministry of Health and registered as the in-charge for the establishment.

The RMI may possess ENDs for pain relief and palliative care & opioid substitution therapy of (OST) as approved by the Drug Commissioner as per estimates of requirement of ENDs.

B. PURCHASE OF ESSENTIAL NARCOTIC DRUGS (ENDs)

1. Thoroughly check your invoice for correct Name and Address of Supplier, Drug License No, Sales Tax No, quantity, batch number and expiry. Original receipt of the consignment of ENDs in the format of Form 3C should be retained for two years and one copy is returned to the supplier and one copy is sent to the State Drugs Controller.

2. Purchase minimum quantity possible.

3. Do not accept these drugs from unauthorized persons or medical representatives or on challan.

4. Accept/Receive supply from the authorized wholesaler/dealer only.

5. Do not accept these drugs as replacement for settlement of expiry or claims.

C. STORAGE AND RECORDS

1. Store all ENDs medicines safely and place them under double lock and key under the supervision of a qualified person or a responsible person.

2. In case of theft or loss, immediately inform the Drugs Control Authorities.

3. Maintain proper records of all sales and purchases for a period of two years. Record of day-to-day accounts of every transactions in END is maintained in the format of Form 3D. Once verified, the doctor-in-charge should sign below the last entry of the day in the register.

   The total quantity possessed by the RMI at any one time should not exceed the submitted estimate (or revised estimate, if any). The revised estimate for ENDs should be submitted by the 31st August along with brief justification. Annual return for the calender year should be filed on or before 31st March in the format of Form 3I.

4. Do not accept any telephonic orders.

5. All expired/damaged stock should be returned by filling in all the relevant details and obtaining stamps/ signatures on the "goods returned" proforma. If sent by transport/ courier, maintain a copy of the proof of delivery or receipt.

D. PRESCRIPTION OF NARCOTIC DRUGS

1. Be completely written in the prescriber's <u>hand writing</u> in ink. Accept electronic prescription only if all applicable requirements are met.

2. Be signed & dated (not computer generated)

3. Carry the prescribers' address (Doctor's full name (and registration no.) address and phone number)

4. Carry the patient's full name, address and, if appropriate, date of birth, if another family member shares the same name.

5. State the form of the drug

6. State the total quantity of the drug or the number of dose units to be disposed in both words & figures including

   i. The name and form of the drug.

   ii. The strength of a preparation (where appropriate)

   iii. The dose to be taken

7. State the exact size of each dose.

8. The total quantity to be supplied in words and figures

9. Prescriptions for ENDs are valid for 14 days only.

10. It is not permitted to prescribe ENDs by the 'repeat' method.

    For details of dispensing see Chapter on Good Dispensing Practices.

E. RESPONSIBILITY OF PHARMACIST

The pharmacist is responsible for:

1. The safe and appropriate management of ENDs in the store:

   i. Ensuring that staff comply with the regulatory requirements and that procedures are in place for the management of ENDs within their area of responsibility.

   ii. Ensuring stock levels of ENDs preparations held in stores.

   iii. Ensuring that their staff, especially new employees, locum staff and agency staff, have access to and adhere to this policy and procedures herein

    iv.   The completion of quarterly observational audit of practice.

2.   The senior Chief/senior pharmacist or pharmacist in-charge is responsible

    i.   For the ENDs key(s) which should be held on their person and separate from all other keys.

    ii.   For keeping the ENDs register up-to-date, accurate and in good order.

    iii.   For ensuring the stock balance of all ENDs entered in the ENDs are checked and reconciled in accordance with the regulatory requirements and Standard Operating Procedure (SOP) of the health facility.

F. ENDs STOCK REGISTER REQUIREMENTS

1.   Be in a bound register (not loose-leaf version)

2.   Each ward/department should have its own ENDs Record Book.

3.   On receipt of all ENDs the pharmacist-in-charge should check the drugs against the requisition and sign the copy of the requisition and immediately record their receipt, including the serial number of the order, in RED ink in the ENDs Record Book.

4.   Entries must be made legibly in chronological order using black ink.

5.   Have separate sections for each class of drug

6.   Show the class of drug at the head of each page

7.   The entry in the ENDs Record Book should state date, time received, drug name and quantity and new stock balance. The stock balance should be checked so that it tallies with the quantity physically present.

8.   Each entry should be countersigned individually. Signing against groups of entries bracketed together must not occur.

9.   Transferring Balances to a New Page or New Record Book

    i.   The balance carried forward should be stated at the top of the new, continuation page so the top line of the new page is not used to record administration to a patient. i.e. date, time, balance carried forward from previous page number, signature & balance.

    ii.   The page number onto which the record is to be continued should be stated at the bottom of the completed page, i.e. 'continued on page "X".

    iii.   Entries should not be made in the space below the last line on any page of the ENDs Record Book.

    iv.   The index should be updated with the new page number

G. ERRORS IN ENTRIES IN THE ENDs RECORD BOOK

1.   No cancellation, obliteration or alteration may be made. It is important that the incorrect entry is readable, therefore, entries should not be scrubbed or tippexed out, obliterated or deleted.

2.   The erroneous entry should be bracketed clearly and marked with an asterisk, the original entry must still be legible. The reason for the error must be indicated by a numbered footnote. This should be signed, dated and witnessed preferably by a second Registered pharmacist or Nurse, or other suitably trained, registered professional.

3.   The correct entry should be made on the next available line. This must be signed and dated.

4.   Be kept on the premises to which the register relates and be available for inspection at any time.

5. Be kept safe for 2 years from the date of the last entry.

H. MANAGING STOCKS OF ENDs

1. Cabinet or safe made of metal with suitable hinges and cabinet fixed to a wall or the floor with rag bolts that are not accessible from outside the cabinet or ENDs locked cupboard that is permanently fixed to the wall. This may be separate from or within another medicines cupboard used to store internal medicines.

2. Before ordering any END check carefully the amount required as END cannot be returned.

3. For pharmacy & clinical areas, including operation theatre and ambulatory services take particular care to ensure sufficient stocks of ENDs for evenings and weekends. Use the handover checks using 5 S as an opportunity to check that stock is sufficient and re-order as required. In this a fixed quantity let's say 10 ampoules of ENDs are taken out (as depicted in the jewellary tray) and the quantity used is immediately replaced to keep the count of 10 for every handover during the change of shifts. Any shortage is immediately noticed thus making accounting easy. For details see chapter on Quality in Quality Tools in Pharmacy and Medical Stores.

Identifies a specific storage space or cell with a corresponding code

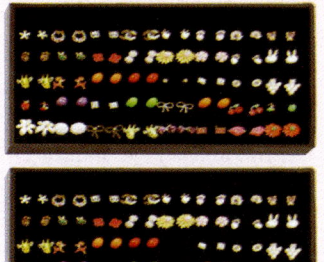

4. Any stock discrepancies must be reported immediately for investigation.

5. An incident form must be completed and the Pharmacy Services Manager be notified.

6. This should include processes for review of environmental security (in particular your own security) and segregation of high strength stock, patient's own ENDs and exposed ENDs.

I. GOLDEN RULES FOR SOPs

1. The pharmacist-in-charge must hold the keys to the ENDs cabinet(s).

2. ENDs keys MUST only be given to a registered pharmacist with delegated authority from the officer-in-charge.

3. Each time a ENDs is removed from the ENDs cabinet, the stock balance of an individual preparation should be confirmed to be correct and the new balance recorded in the ENDs Record Book.

4. A record MUST be made in the ENDs when a ENDs is removed from the ENDs cabinet and issued.

5. At each point where a ENDs moves from the authorized possession of one person to another, the transfer should be recorded by means of the signatures of both parties.

6. The stock balance of all ENDs recorded in the ENDs Register must be checked at each change of shift with the minimum of a daily check. using 5 S tool (for details see section on quality tools in pharmacy and medical stores). Potential approaches to reducing the risk of diversion include:

    i. Use of automated medication dispensing systems.

    ii. Restricting the supply in ward stocks (e.g. codeine, dihydrocodeine, zopiclone, diazepam) by having smaller stock holdings but more frequent pharmacy 'top-ups'.

    iii. Checking for discrepancies in stock balances at shift handover (described as above).

iv.   Local reclassification to a more strictly controlled schedule (e.g., managing alprazolam/diazepam as controlled drug rather than Schedule H1 that must meet storage and register requirements).

v.   Close monitoring of repeat prescriptions.

J. MANAGING ROUTINE OVERAGE OR UNDERAGE FOR LIQUID ENDs

1.   Liquid ENDs can often be marginally out due to small but repeated errors in the measuring process. This can be reduced by using the smallest measuring device possible e.g., oral syringes for lower doses.

2.   Write the overage/underage quantity in the ENDs register clearly marked as overage/underage by the reconciler, signed and dated.

3.   The stock identified as overage can be returned to the container and used for subsequent supplies/administrations.

4.   Any unexpected increase in the overage/underage should be considered and managed as a discrepancy.

K. MISSING ENDs AND KEYS

1.   If the ENDs keys cannot be found then urgent efforts should be made to retrieve the keys as speedily as possible e.g., by contacting staff who have just gone off duty. The Senior pharmacist or Chief Pharmacist or Management should be informed as soon as possible. Depending on the circumstances, it may also be appropriate to contact the police.

2.   An incident Report form (IR) should be completed.

Procedure for missing ENDs

3.   Inform all staff about missing ENDs.

4.   Enter the time and date of the discovery of the missing drug on the appropriate page.

5.   The discrepancy must be investigated and resolved without delay. It is important to remember that a discrepancy may indicate misuse. Report discrepancy to a senior pharmacist within one working day. Conduct spot check count of all ENDs stocked. Carefully check transactions in the register and in the stock control system to trace an error or omission.

6.   Record following details:

i.   The exact nature of the stock balance discrepancy.

ii.   Steps taken (both by pharmacist and nurse present) to investigate as above.

iii.   Note when the last balance was signed as being correct.

7.   If an error is traced then a register entry should be made, clearly stating the reason for the entry, the reference of the error or the omission, the date of the error or omission and the signature of both the person carrying out the amendment and the witness. For details see point G above.

8.   If no error or omission can be traced a clinical incident report (IR) should be completed and the Chief Pharmacist and Accountable Officer informed.

9.   The Narcotic Drug procedure should be reminded to all staff.

L. RECORDING BREAKAGE AND WASTAGE OF ENDs

1.   In case of accidental breakage, enter into the Register as with the procedure for giving the drug.

2. Record 'Broken Vial' on the appropriate page, and the entry should be signed by the practitioner who broke the vial and another staff member.

3. When these occur a brief explanation should be stated e.g. if a 2.5mg dose is given from a 5mg ampoule, write 2.5mg given, 2.5mg wasted in the amount given column. If patient refusal results in wastage of the dose, write 'dose refused'.

4. There must be two signatures. Both staff must then proceed to discard the broken vial into a sharps container.

M. TRANSPORT OF ENDs

1. Transport ENDs may be delivered to the authorized ward/ department by a messenger, in a locked box or a sealed, tamper evident container, provided that a signature is obtained on the appropriate document each time the package changes hands.

2. Upon delivery to the ward/ department the package should be handed to the Nurse-in-charge, who is an authorized signatory for ENDs. This must be a Registered Nurse. The Nurse should sign to acknowledge receipt.

3. The messenger must be an authorized staff and should be wearing an ID badge.

4. On no account should ENDs be left unattended.

N. TRANSFER OF WARDS

1. When a ward is being transferred, all ENDs should be checked against the Record Book and put into a box along with the ENDs Record Book and the ENDs Ordering Book.

2. This should be carried out by the nurse-in-charge of the ward along with a second witness.

3. The box must be locked and sealed then stored in the pharmacy until the ward reopens.

4. The Registered Nurse-in-charge of opening the ward is responsible for opening the box. All the drugs must be checked by the Registered nurse and a witness and then returned to the ward ENDs cupboard. When the ward re-opens it is the responsibility of the Matron to produce an up-to-date list of authorized signatures for the pharmacy department.

O. ENDs BROUGHT IN BY PATIENTS

1. Patients' own ENDs remain their property during their in-patient stay, however they should not routinely be stored on the ward. Whenever possible they should be returned to the patient's relatives to be taken home. If the ENDs are no longer required they may, with the patient's permission be destroyed as set out in SOP. The permission should be documented in the notes and the ENDs stored temporarily as described below.

2. Temporary storage of patients' own ENDs on the ward may be necessary whilst they are awaiting collection and removal to the pharmacy or to the patient's home. In this situation, they should be placed in the ENDs cupboard but should be clearly marked and kept separate from ward stock.

3. Patients' own ENDs should not be used during the admission except in an emergency. If they are used, they must only be administered to the patient to whom they belong.

4. A full record (with double signed entries) of the patient's own ENDs being held should be kept on a separate page at the back of the ENDs Record Book. They must be signed out from the ENDs Record Book when returned.

5. A space of six lines should be left under an entry of an individual patient's ENDs, a separate page should be used for each entry.

6. Patient's own drugs should not be included in the stock balance but should still be counted and recorded in the daily check. The drugs should be returned to the patient on their discharge, at which time they should be signed out from the ENDs Record Book and signed by a Registered Nurse and a witness (preferably by a second Registered Nurse, or other suitably trained, Registered professional).

P. DISPOSAL OF ENDs

All facilities disposing of ENDs, all care must be taken to ensure that they are not open to abuse, stocks awaiting destruction are separated and stored separately.

1. Expired or unwanted controlled drugs cannot be returned.

2. Separate expired stock from the current stock and clearly labelled as "expired, unwanted stock/excess stock or suspected illicit substance awaiting destruction" in order to minimize the risk of error and inadvertent supply to patients.

3. Note in the daily count record book the details of which stock and the amount is due for destruction. NOTE these items must still be counted daily until destroyed.

4. Do not delete items from the ENDs register until it is actually destroyed.

5. The store-in-charge should arrange an appointment for the destruction of the items by an authorized person.

6. Disposal of ENDs should be done in the presence of an authorised officer nominated by the State Drugs Controller.

7. Follow manufacturer's instructions for disposal carefully.

8. The ENDs quarantined for destruction should be added to the denaturing kit according to the process below:

   i. Order of adding products to kit: solid oral dose forms (e.g., tablets/capsules, suspected illicit solids), powder containing injection, and transdermal patches, small volume liquids e.g., injection ampoules, large volume liquids e.g., oral liquids.

   ii. Processing products before adding to kit:

      a. Tablets and capsules should be removed from all packaging.

      b. Injection ampoules/vials should be opened and the contents and glass added to the contents.

      c. Transdermal patches should be cut in two.

   iii. Liquids should be emptied from the container and the container rinsed with a small volume of water.

   iv. Add water, as necessary, in accordance with the manufacturer's instructions

   v. The liquid contents of opened or partly used ampoules should be placed into a black lidded burn bin. This also applies to discontinued or partly used patient controlled analgesia (PCA) epidural or solutions in syringe drivers.

   vi. Fold used patches and place in a black lidded burn bin.

   vii. Oral ENDs dispensed but refused by a patient should be placed in a black lidded burn bin with some liquid soap.

   viii. Destruction process must be witnessed by a second person.

ix. If there are a large number of items being destroyed, the inactivation process may take up to 24 hours for the process to complete; in this case the used kit should then be put in the ENDs cupboard whilst the inactivation process is taking place. The ENDs are now considered 'irretrievable' and the responsibility of the authorised witness is complete. Note: the kit contents will form a gel within a few minutes and may become hot initially (this is normal). The used kit should be disposed of as medicinal waste for incineration in a sharps bin (yellow lid yellow body).

x. Do not place in a clinical waste bag.

9. Write-off the ENDs of the ENDs record book as they are destroyed. The entry must specify: the date, time and location, the name, strength and form of the drug, quantity destroyed followed by a printed name, signature professional status alongside the printed name, professional status and signature of the authorised witness.

10. Make a note of the drugs destroyed on the ENDs destruction record sheet. There must be two signatures.

11. Reconcile the remaining ENDs stock.

Q. MANAGEMENT OF ENDs SPILLAGES AND PART USED DOSES

Spillages should be managed according to the Spills Management Policy as below:

1. Spillages must be cleaned up quickly, wearing gloves. The spillages should be soaked up with paper towel, taking care not to puncture the skin from broken glass or needles. The soaked paper towel should be disposed off in the sharps bin as medicinal waste for incineration. This procedure is followed by thorough cleaning with neutral detergent and water.

2. Spillages on the skin should be washed with soap and water. If drugs are splashed into the eyes irrigate with water or sterile 0.9% normal saline. Seek medical or occupational health advice. The details of the spillage should be documented in the ENDs register and initialed by the person who made the spillage and preferably a second registered nurse or other registered practitioner.

3. The pharmacist/authorized person doing the 3 monthly checks should note any spillages on the comments section of the checks. Tablets/capsules dropped on the floor should be put in a clearly labelled and sealed envelope stating the reason and treated as expired stock.

4. Doses of ENDs that are prepared but not administered or only partly used must be destroyed immediately by being emptied into the sharps bin in the ward/department by a Registered Nurse and witnessed by a second Registered Nurse.

5. Record details of the amount given to the patient and the amount destroyed in the ENDs register.

Audit relating to different aspects of the ENDs SOPs should be carried out at regular intervals as part of the annual medicines management audit.

Common problems observed with handling of ENDs are:

- Named persons not responsible for ENDs keys at all times
- Potential theft of ENDs by using missing ENDs keys.
- ENDs not stored correctly
- Records not kept as required
- Signatures not obtained on delivery

- Failure to take ENDs from patients on admission
- ENDs not separated for destruction appropriately (potential for administration)
- Record not made of ENDs awaiting destruction.
- Inaccurate ENDs register entry.
- Failure to complete ENDs register entries
- Denaturing kit not available
- Failure to use denaturing kit as per manufacturers instructions. Used denaturing kits not collected in an appropriate and timely manner
- ENDs stock destroyed in the absence of an authorized witness
- Failure to complete ENDs destruction record

12 | Security and Protection of Stores

Like any other valuable items, medicines can also be stolen too. Not only this, some people who are addicted to various drugs and try to steal certain medicines. Security breaches include theft, bribery, and fraud and can be substantial with disastrous economic and health effects. To safeguard medicines, avoid expensive losses, and prevent unnecessary drug abuse in the masses, medical stores need to be protected.

I. SECURITY OF STORES

A. PROTECT EQUIPMENT

Most medical stores today have basic equipment and electronics such as laptop or computer and barcode scanner machine, etc. These equipment and electronics are constantly at the risk of damage or burglary. Thus, to prevent equipment from any physical or information theft, it is important to secure the store with high-end security systems.

B. SECURE THE STAFF AND CUSTOMERS

The staff and customers of a medical store should feel secure when they are inside the store. The medical store owner or manager is ideally responsible for their safety and security. The criminals may attack and injure your staff and customers. Therefore, the store must be secured with video surveillance and alarm systems. Security for medical stores often includes panic buttons for an unforeseen event.

C. SECURE PHARMACEUTICALS

1. During transport
   i. Verify documents.
   ii. Ensure packing seals are used.
   iii. Use strong boxes/containers.
   iv. Provide reliable/well-maintained vehicles.
   v. Ensure drivers are reliable.
   vi. Ensure rapid clearance at air and sea ports and through on-land borders.
2. At storage facilities
   i. Limit access to designated staff only.
   ii. Limit the number of keys made for the facility; keep a list of people who have keys.
   iii. Secure all locks and doors.
   iv. Make unannounced spot checks.
   v. Provide independent periodic stock count/inventory control.

3. In health centres
    i. Lock the storeroom/cupboards.
    ii. Maintain inventory control cards for each product.
    iii. Set maximum dispensing quantities especially for reserve, expensive, scheduled drugs.
    iv. Keep record of individual prescriptions and maintain prescription or dispensing registers as deemed necessary.
    v. Limit dispensing to authorize staff members only.

D. THEFT PREVENTION AND CONTROL

1. Providing unique identifiers for all pharmaceutical supplies.
2. Controlling access to the storage facility to authorized personnel only.
3. Review of security measures and closing of sources and outlets of theft.
4. Improving record keeping and maintaining a perpetual inventory control system.
5. Monitor select products
    i. As additional protection against theft, monitor items that are fast moving, chronically in short supply, in high demand by patients (hence a good open market for the product), expensive, life saving, and easy to hide or disguise due to weak security measures.
    ii. Select medicines likely to be stolen or misused (e.g., antibiotics, narcotics, psychotropic agents, antiretroviral, etc.).
    iii. Check inventory records for stock on hand. Then, conduct a physical inventory (physically count the quantities on hand) and compare the results.
    iv. Check the inventory records to determine the consumption during a specified period. Then, check medical charts or prescription ledgers and count the number of treatment courses during the same period. Convert treatment courses into dose units and compare this figure with the stock issued from the storage area.
    v. If you find a significant discrepancy, investigate further.
6. It is incumbent upon the responsible store in-charge/pharmacist to inform relevant authorities whenever instances of theft of pharmaceutical products are discovered.

II. PROTECTING AGAINST FIRE

To prevent damage to products from fire:

1. Ensure adequate signages in the pharmacy of medical store (see below).
2. Make standard fire extinguishers available in every storage facility according to national regulations. The design should meet the local building codes and the requirements of insurers in respect of
    i. Accessibility to fire department
    ii. Adequate escape routes and emergency doors with locks that do not prevent staff from leaving the building in emergency
    iii. Compartmentalize building/ storage of flammables to reduce the risk of fire.
3. Visually inspect fire extinguishers every 2-3 months to ensure that pressures are maintained and the extinguisher is ready for use. Service fire extinguishers at least every 12 months.

4. Place smoke detectors and sprinkles throughout the storage facility and check them every 2-3 months to ensure that they are working properly.

5. Strictly prohibit smoking in the store.

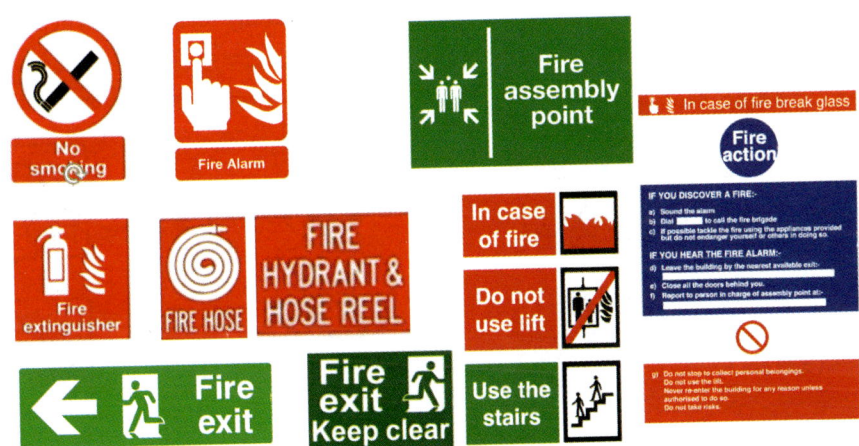

6. Conduct fire drills for personnel every 6 months.

7. Clearly mark emergency exits and check regularly to be sure they are not blocked or inaccessible.

8. Display fire precaution signs in appropriate places in the storage facility (especially in locations where flammables are stored).

9. Use sand to extinguish fires where there are no fire extinguishers. Place buckets of sand near the door.

10. Four main types of fire extinguishers:

   i. **Dry chemical** extinguishers contain an extinguishing agent such as potassium bicarbonate (similar to baking soda), and use a compressed gas as a propellant. They are effective for multiple types of fire including combustible solids like wood or paper, combustible liquids like gasoline or grease, and electrical fires.

   ii. **Water** extinguishers contain water and compressed gas and should only be used on ordinary combustibles, such as paper and wood. Never use water on fires caused by liquids (such as gasoline or kerosene) or electrical fires.

   iii. **Carbon dioxide (CO_2)** extinguishers are most effective on fires caused by liquids (such as gasoline or kerosene) and electrical fires, but not on fires caused by combustibles like paper, cardboard, or lumber. The gas disperses quickly and does not leave any harmful residue.

   iv. **Halon** extinguishers are often used in areas with computer equipment or other machinery because they leave no residue. They can be used on common combustibles, flammable liquids, and electrical fires. However, halon is dangerous to inhale and harmful to the environment. They are most effective in confined spaces, but remember that the area will need to be ventilated before it can be reoccupied.

11. Be sure medical store staff are trained in how to use fire extinguishers.

12. RACE and PASS are simple methods used to teach and use of fire extinguisher (see below):

The PASS method is accepted for dry chemical and carbon dioxide (CO_2) extinguishers; however, other methods are needed when using water and other extinguishers and with special fires, such as flammable liquids. Additionally, the PASS method may not be appropriate for all dry chemical and CO_2 extinguishers. Be sure to carefully read the instructions for the extinguishers in your facility.

Remember the RACE word (Healthcare fire safety)

Rescue anyone in immediate danger of the fire.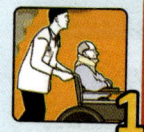

Alarm Pull the nearest fire alarm and call fire response.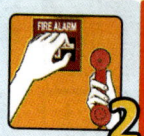

Contain fire by closing all door in the fire area.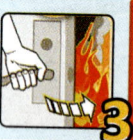

Extinguish small fires. If not, leave the area and close the door.

Remember the PASS word to operate Fire extinguisher

Pull Pull the pin (or other motion) to unlock the extinguisher.

Aim Aim at the base (bottom)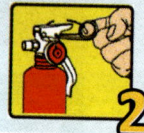

Squeeze Squeeze the lever.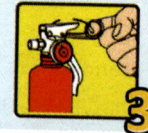

Sweep Sweep the spray from left to right.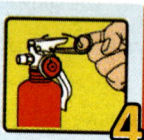

III. PROTECTING AGAINST PESTS

1. Prevention inside the storage facility

   i. Design or modify the storeroom to facilitate cleaning and prevent moisture.

   ii. Maintain a clean environment to prevent conditions that favour pests. For example, store garbage in covered garbage bins. Regularly clean floors and shelves.

   iii. Do not store or leave food in the storage facility.

   iv. Keep the interior of the building as dry as possible.

   v. Paint or varnish wood, as needed.

   vi. Use pallets and shelving.

   vii. Prevent pests from entering the facility.

   viii. Inspect the storage facility regularly for evidence of pests.

   ix. Packaging and shipping cartons can be treated to prevent pest infestation. For example, cartons can be shrink-wrapped or non-toxic desiccating (dehydrating) agents can be added.

2. Prevention outside the storage facility

   i. Regularly inspect and clean the outside premises of the storage facility, especially areas where garbage is stored. Check for any rodent burrows, and be sure that garbage and other waste is stored in covered containers.

ii. Check for still or stagnant pools of water in and around the premises, and be sure that there are no buckets, old tires, or other items holding water.

iii. Treat wood frame facilities with water sealant, as needed.

iv. Use mercury vapour lighting where possible, and locate lighting away from the building to minimize the attraction of pests.

3. **Strategies for specific pests**

   i. **Rodents:** Rodent problems are best solved by prohibiting rodent entry and maintaining a dry, clean facility. Other alternatives include—traditional, spring-loaded snap traps baited with food; glue boards, which are disposable plastic or wood trays partially filled with nontoxic, adhesive glue; bait boxes, which are shoe-sized boxes with lids and holes on each end containing toxic rodenticide packets; electronic ultrasonic devices, which emit high- frequency sounds, causing rodents to avoid the area; or rat poison.

   ii. **Birds or bats:** If the facility has space between the ceiling and the roof, cover all the openings with fine wire mesh to prevent birds or bats from entering the storeroom.

   iii. **Flying pests:** The best prevention is to keep all doors and windows of the storage facility closed or screened off from the outside. Make sure there are no holes in the walls, floor, or ceiling. Insect electrocuting light traps ("bug zappers," hanging electric grids that attract flying insects via a bright fluorescent or ultraviolet light) may be appropriate in some situations. However, they should be placed away from supplies, since ultraviolet light damages a number of products (especially latex products, such as a male condoms).

   iv. **Reptiles:** Most snake species are innocuous and can be managed with noisemakers and by keeping the outside of the facility clear of bushes. If snakes are an especially difficult problem in your area, you can construct a snake-proof fence around the perimeter of the facility. The fence should be made with heavy, galvanized screen with 6 mm wire mesh. The fence should be 90 cm tall with the lower end buried at least 10-16 cm in the ground. The above ground portion of the fence should be slanted at a 30° angel outward from the base and away from the building, using supporting stakes inside the fence.

   Strategies for reptiles

   30°

   90 cm

   10–16 cm

   v. **Termites/structural pests:** There are two primary treatments for termites, but both are expensive and require a specialist. The first treatment involves injecting a termiticide into the soil in the ground beneath the facility. If the problem is severe, or if the first treatment is not feasible, the building must be fumigated. All stored goods must be removed from the site during fumigation. Replace wood severely damaged by structural pests.

4. **There are alternative methods of controlling structural pests**

   i. Use nontoxic heat or liquid nitrogen treatments.

   ii. Build metal barriers into the foundation of a new building. Sheets of metal protrude from between the foundation and walls of the building. The sheets are bent downward at an angle, but not touching the ground. When termites or ants attempt to climb up the foundation, they encounter the metal barrier that they cannot climb around.

   Construct sand barriers around the building as a preventative measure. However, the grains of sand must be a specific size, and this method can be expensive.

13 | Handling of Expired or Damaged Stock, and their Safe Disposal

Storage facility grounds, including the area around health centers, must remain free of health care waste and other garbage. Maintaining a clean environment where pharmaceuticals and other health supplies are stored will reduce the number of pests-insects and rodents- and reduce the number of people, including children, who may be injured by used medical equipment or discarded medicines. Incorrect management of waste places waste handlers, health workers and the community at risk of infection and injury.

Plan storage, transportation, and disposal techniques that are practical and simple. Monitor disposal practices on a regular, frequent basis.

I. TYPES OF WASTE AND THEIR DISPOSAL METHOD

Different types of waste that must be destroyed safely and effectively and their methods of disposal include-

Non-medical waste

Garden rubbish: Compost leaves, sticks, weeds, and trimmings from shrubs and trees, if feasible. Designate a separate area for composting.

Cardboard cartons: If possible, recycle cardboard; otherwise, treat like ordinary rubbish.

Ordinary rubbish: Where municipal solid waste facilities exist, dispose of ordinary rubbish in the municipal dump. Otherwise, bury it.

Human waste: Use pit latrines or other toileting facilities to dispose of all human waste.

Health care waste

Sharps waste: Single-use disposable needles, needles from auto-disable syringes, scalpel blades, sharp instruments requiring disposal, and sharps waste from laboratory procedures.

Other hazardous medical waste: Waste contaminated with blood, body fluids, human tissue; compounds such as mercury; pressurized containers; and wastes with high heavy metal content.

Pharmaceuticals: Expired, damaged, or otherwise unusable medicines and items contaminated by or containing medicinal substances.

II. HANDLING OF PRODUCTS DECLARED AS NOT-OF-STANDARD-QUALITY

Follow institutional policy. Preferably, products declared as not-of-standard–quality (NSQ) should not be returned to the manufacturer.

They should be clearly labeled as not for use, segregated and competent authorities, states drug regulatory authority and the supplier of the product should be informed.

Herewith products declared as NSQ should be handled as for expired medicines. These items should be written off the record as per the guidelines of the Institution and disposed as per Bio-medical Waste (Management & Handling) Rules, 2016 and amendments.

III. SAFE DISPOSAL AND DESTRUCTION

Why safe disposal is important?

Most expired medicines become less efficacious and few may be toxic, but the defective disposal of them poses serious threat to the public health. Of special concern is the inappropriate disposal of large quantities of antibiotics, steroids, antidepressants, analgesics, anticancer drugs and many more. Improper disposal of antibiotics has been identified as one of the contributing factors to the emergence of antimicrobial resistance. Return to the manufacturer wherever feasible should be the first choice because the manufacturer is likely to have good disposal method at its disposal. However, be aware of possible pilfering from a stockpile of waste drugs may result in expired drugs being diverted to the market for resale and misuse as incident described above. Expired medicines may come into the hands of scavengers and children, if a landfill is insecure.

Some of the issues relating to the inappropriate disposal of expired medicines are:

- Possibility of contaminating drinking water source or supply from the disposal place the leachate may get access to the water supply system.

- Disposal of non-biodegradable antibiotics, anti-neoplastics and disinfectants into the sewage system may kill bacteria necessary for treatment of sewage. Flushing of anti-neoplastics into water resource may damage aquatic life or contaminate drinking water. Discharge of large amount of undiluted disinfectants into the sewage system or water resources may too cause similar situation.

- Burning of the expired medicines at low temperature or in open containers results in release of toxic pollutants to the air. Ideally this should be avoided.

- Inefficient and insecure disposal may lead to recycling of the expired medicines. This is true especially when they are disposed in original containers.

Safe Handling of Waste

1. Drug store facilities require a sound waste drug handling system to minimize damage to health and the environment caused by their wasted drugs.

2. A written wasted drugs management plan describing all the practices for handling, storing, treating, and disposing of hazardous and non-hazardous waste, as well as types of worker training should be drawn up after doing a comprehensive assessment of waste handling at the facility.

3. Clearly assign staff responsibilities. Make responsibilities clear so that workers feel accountable for how well tasks are completed and so that no step in the process is overlooked.

4. Written internal rules for generation, handling, storage, treatment, and disposal. Formalize desired practices, as written rules may be better maintained.

5. Managing health care waste is a comprehensive programme that requires support at all levels of the health care system. Staff involved in health care waste management must be given training and support in safe handling, storage, treatment, and disposal of pharmaceuticals. Training is necessary to ensure that staff are aware of all hazards they might meet and that they are practicing good hygiene, safe sharps handling, proper use of protective clothing, proper packaging and labelling of waste, and safe storage of waste.

6. Protective Equipment (PPE) availability: Workers need specific types of PPE, such as surgical masks and gloves, aprons, and boots, to protect themselves when moving and treating various types of wasted drugs.

7. Good hygiene practices: Many infectious agents must enter the mouth or be swallowed to cause disease. Even if protective PPE is worn, some organisms will get on workers' hands and faces. Thus, workers need to wash their hands and faces regularly with soap and warm water.

8. Vaccination of workers against potentially deadly viral hepatitis B and tetanus infections.

9. Temporary storage containers in designated locations: Hazardous healthcare wastes should be stored only for short periods—not more than 72 hours in the warm season in warm climates. Also, they should be put in a labelled, covered container in a fixed location—for example, a specific corner of the room.

10. Minimization, reuse, and recycling procedures: The less waste generated, the less there is to manage. Unnecessary disposal of valuable chemicals and pharmaceuticals can be avoided through good inventory practices: for example, by using the oldest batch first by never opening a new container before the last one is finished; by preventing products from being thrown out during routine cleaning; and by checking on delivery to make sure materials are not about to expire.

11. A waste segregation system: Segregating (sorting and separating) wasted drugs both reduces the volume of waste and enables different kinds of materials to be handled appropriately

12. Treatment methods for hazardous and highly hazardous waste. Identifying and training responsible staff are a first step in the effective management of wasted drugs.

13. Expired drugs found in the distribution network should be kept apart from other medicinal products to avoid any confusion. They should be clearly labelled as not-for-use and competent authorities and supplier of the product should be informed.

14. Take non-usable and expired medications off the shelf and store in a separate, secure area under the control of pharmacy, until final disposal. Hazardous, toxic substances and flammable materials should be stored in suitably designed and segregated, enclosed areas in conformity with Central, State Legislations and SOPs.

15. Expired medicines should be written off the record as per the guidelines of the Institution.

16. Ensure that out-of-date stock procedure is followed by clearly marking them in black and segregate them from in-date stock, until out-of-date stock destroyed.

17. All expired pharmaceuticals should be destroyed as per the provisions of the Bio-Medical Waste (Management and Handling) Rules, 2016 and its amendments. (For details see section below).

IV. DISPOSAL METHODS

1. Burial pits and encapsulation are suitable in locations without shallow groundwater and for small volumes of waste.

    i. **Burial pits:** The bottom of the pit should be 1.5 m above the groundwater level, 3-5 m deep, and lined with a substance of low permeability, such as clay. Surround the opening with a mound to keep run-off water from entering the hole, and build a fence around the area. Periodically, cover waste layers with 10-15 cm of soil.

    ii. **Encapsulation:** Cement-lined pits or high-density plastic containers or drums are filled to 75% capacity with health care waste. The container is then filled with plastic foam, sand, cement, or clay to immobilize the waste. The encapsulated waste is then disposed of in a landfill or left in place if the container is constructed in the ground.

    iii. **Incineration:** Medium- and high-temperature incineration devices require a capital investment and an operations and maintenance budget. They operate on fuel, wood, or other combustible material and produce solid ashes and gases. Pollutants are emitted to varying degrees. The ash is toxic and must be buried in a protected pit. Combustible waste is reduced to incombustible waste with a decreased volume. The high temperatures kill microorganisms.

Medium-temperature incinerators, commonly a double-chamber design or pyrolytic incinerator, operate at a medium-temperature combustion process (800°- 1,000°C).

High-temperature incinerators, recommended by WHO, treat health care waste at a temperature >1,000°C.

2. When operated by staff trained in correct use and maintenance, incineration-

    i. Completely destroys needles and syringes

    ii. Kills microorganisms

    iii. Reduces the volume of waste

    iv. Generates less air pollution than low-temperature burning.

    Note: Incinerate pharmaceuticals only, if absolutely necessary.

3. **Low-temperature burning:** Burning devices not exceeding 400° C include single-chamber brick hearths, drum burners, and burning pits. They burn incompletely and do not fully destroy waste. They may not kill microorganisms, given these shortcomings; low temperature burning should be used only as a short-term solution.

4. **Burn and bury:** Pit burning is a low-cost but relatively ineffective means of waste disposal. A fence should surround the pit to prevent children, animals, and others from coming into contact with the waste. The pit location should avoid walking paths (high-traffic areas). The fire, usually started with a petroleum-based fuel and allowed to burn, should be supervised by designated staff and located down-wind of the facility and residential areas. The low-temperature fire emits pollutants, and the ash and remaining material should be covered with 10-15 cm of dirt.

5. **Safety boxes**

    Safety boxes or sharps containers are puncture- and water-resistant, impermeable containers. When used correctly, they reduce the risk of skin-puncture injuries that may spread disease.

    i. Do not recap syringes before disposal.

    ii. Place the syringe and needle in the sharps box **immediately** after use.

    iii. Keep the sharps box where the injections are given.

    iv. Do not overfill the sharps containers (about ¾ full).

    v. When ¾ full, close box tab completely to cover the opening and tape it shut.

    vi. Store the box in a safe and secure location until ready for final disposal.

    vii. Do not empty and refill sharp boxes. Fill once and discard immediately.

6. **Other method:** In addition to the common methods, other methods are used in some setting, including needle removal/needle destruction, melting syringes, steam sterilization (autoclaving and hydro-claving), and micro-waving (with shredding).

7. **Waste types NOT to be incinerated**

    i. Pressurized gas containers.

    ii. Large amounts of reactive chemical waste.

    iii. Silver salts and photographic or radiographic wastes.

    iv. Halogenated plastics such as polyvinyl chloride (PVC).

    v.   Waste with high mercury or cadmium content, such as broken thermometers, used batteries, and lead-lined wooden panels.

   vi.   Sealed ampoules or ampoules containing heavy metals.

8.   The disposal methods for various categories of pharmaceuticals are identified in the Table below. For disposal of hazardous drugs see section on Hazardous Drugs.

9.   Particular attention must be given to disposal of the following categories of pharmaceuticals:

- Controlled substances, such as narcotics and psychotropic medicines.
- Anti-infective drugs
- Antineoplastics
- Cytotoxics anti-cancer drugs, toxic drugs
- Antiseptics and disinfectants

Disposal methods for various categories of pharmaceuticals.

CATEGORY	DISPOSAL METHODS	COMMENTS
Solids **Semi-solids** **Powders**	Landfill Waste encapsulation Waste inertization Medium and high temperature incineration (cement kiln incinerator)	No more than 1% of the daily municipal waste should be disposed of daily in an untreated from (non-immobilized) to a landfill.
Liquids	Sewer High temperature incineration (cement kiln incinerator)	Antineoplastics—not to sewer
Ampoules	Crush ampoules and flush diluted fluid to sewer	Antineoplastics—not to sewer
Anti-infective drugs	Waste encapsulation Waste inertization Medium and high temperature incineration (cement kiln incinerator)	Liquid antibiotics may be diluted with water, left to stand for several weeks and discharged to a sewer
Antineoplastics	Return to donor or manufacturer Waste encapsulation Waste inertization Medium and high temperature incineration (cement kiln incinerator) (chemical decomposition)	Not to landfill unless encapsulated Not to sewer No medium temperature Incineration.
Narcotics and Psychotropic Drugs	Waste encapsulation Waste inertization Medium and high temperature incineration (cement kiln incinerator)	Not to landfill unless encapsulated.
Aerosol canister	Landfill Waste encapsulation	Not to be burnt: may explode.
Disinfectants	Use To sewer or fast-flowing watercourse: small quantities of diluted disinfectants (max. 50 liters per day under supervision)	No undiluted disinfectants to sewers or water courses. Maximum 50 liters per day diluted to sewer or fast-flowing watercourse. No disinfectants at all to slow moving or stagnant water courses.
PVC plastic, glass	Landfill	Not for burning in open containers.
Paper, cardboard	Recycle, burn, landfill	

14 | Setting up a Medical Store/ Warehouse

The efficiency, effective utilization, running costs, working environment of the medical store or warehouse all depend on its fitness for purpose. Warehouses are expensive investments, therefore, while designing a new warehouse make sure that it does not outgrow its volumetric capacity (quantities of products to be stored) or throughput capacity (incoming goods, customer orders, inter-facility transfers, dispatches and returns) too quickly.

The purpose of the warehouse is to determine its size, physical design, its proportion of indoor warehousing versus outside yard space, its location, dimensions and structural composition, along with provisions for specialized equipment installations and division between storage and working spaces to comfortably hold stocks. It is not desirable that warehouse to be running at 100% of physical capacity, a fair amount of working space is required besides storage space.

I. CONSTRUCTING A MEDICAL STORE

When constructing a medical store, consider the following:

1. **Location:** The store must be accessible to all the health facilities or units to be served. Ideally, a medical store should be located by itself on a separate lot to enhance security and minimize human and automobile congestion. Ensure road access for the largest vehicle that might ever need to come to the store. Do not build the store close to trees with big roots. This can kill the tree, and conversely, trees with aggressive root systems can damage the building's foundation. Also see section on supply chain management and distribution of pharmaceuticals.

2. **Accessibility:** Locate the store so that supplies can be easily received and distributed. This can be near an airport, or near the national road or canal system.

3. **Temperature control:** In temperate climate Air conditioned stores should be designed, and cooling plant sized, so as to ensure that internal temperatures can reliably be maintained below 25⁰C. Entrance to air-conditioned stores should have airlock lobbies, ideally with two sets of self closing flexible doors, so as to minimize loss of cooled air.

   Uncooled stores should be well ventilated; temperature stratification should be reduced by use of ceiling fans or carefully designed natural ventilation. Building should be designed to minimize dust infiltration.

4. **Shading:** Locate the store in an area where trees can be planted to provide shade and offset high temperatures.

5. **Trees:** Although it is ideal to have trees planted for shade, check the condition of any trees already on the site regularly. Cut down any weak trees so they do not fall on the building during inclement (unpleasantly cold or wet) weather. Trim the other trees to avoid falling branches.

6. **Drainage:** Build the store on a raised foundation to allow rainwater to drain away from the store. If possible, locate the store in an area on higher ground.

7. **Security:** Provide the store with adequate security from thieves, fire, etc. Fencing or perimeter walls are often used to improve security and control access.

   i. Unsupervised access from the loading bay to the store itself should not be possible. The main storage area where order picking takes place needs to be very secure.

   ii. Ideally, the office area should have windows over-looking the loading bays and the warehouse access.

   iii. The staff rest area, sanitary facilities, and changing rooms should not have direct access to the warehouse or from the outside.

   iv. Visitors should have separate sanitary facilities.

   v. Staff parking should be well separated from the loading area.

   vi. Adequate perimeter fencing and external lighting should be provided.

II. DESIGNING A MEDICAL STORE

Consider the following when designing a storage facility:

1. **Capacity/space:** Storage facilities must have the capacity for both storage and handling. Ideally, space should be evenly divided between the two. New products and packaging innovations, as well as an increase in products related to the prevention and treatment of disease like HIV/AIDS, malaria, tuberculosis, and hepatitis B, have increased the volume of products and medical consumables that flow through warehouses. This includes items such as bed nets and insecticides for preventing malaria and more medicines to treat TB because of the increase number of TB cases due to HIV/AIDS. When designing a new facility, do not underestimate the storage requirements.

2. **Design of the Warehouse/Medical Store for Growth**

   Wherever possible a warehouse should be designed to allow one-way flow and for future growth, both anticipated and unforeseen. Free movement has priority over storage capacity. Plan for both peak and average conditions and provide plans for future growth. Different layouts can be extended in ways that produce different effects; Sometimes accessibility is improved and sometimes capacity is expanded. It is necessary to know in advance what is required of the extension, and to choose a layout that gives the desired method of expansion whilst minimizing disturbance to the operation. Involve the warehouse employees to get their first hand ideas on the best layout options. Possible layouts are shown below:

   Feature of *T-shaped warehouse* are:

   i. Inward and outward flows are on the same side of building.

   ii. The warehouse can be extended both rearwards and laterally without disruption.

   iii. Inward and outward movement of goods can be monitored from one point.

   Features of *Through Flow warehouse* are:

   i. Inward and outward supplies movement are on opposite sides of the building. Separate staff for monitoring inward and outward movement of supplies is required.

   ii. The building can only be extended sideways without disrupting operations. Provides more storage capacity but reduced accessibility.

   Features of *Corner warehouse* are:

   i. Inward supplies movement and outward supplies movement are on different side of the building. However, movement on both corners can be monitored by one person between the two loading areas.

ii. The warehouse can be extended in two directions in the same way as with the T-shaped plan.

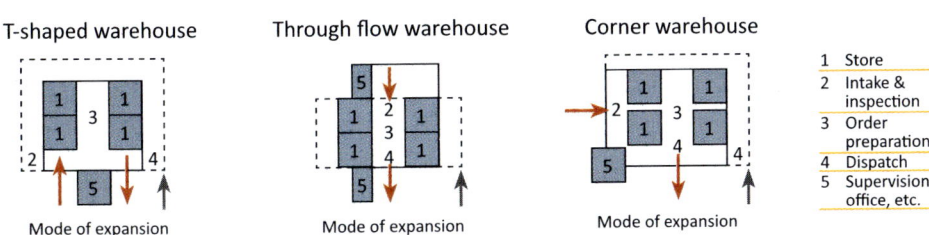

Warehouse and layout principles

3. **Ancillary Accommodation and Loading Bays**

   The design and sizing of ancillary accommodations should be carefully considered. These spaces include offices, staff rooms (for rest, recreation, and eating), sanitary facilities, changing rooms, receiving and packing areas, the vehicle loading bay is a particularly important area. It is essential that it be protected from the weather and big enough to receive the maximum number of vehicles expected at any one time. In larger stores, the loading bay should be raised so that the floor of the vehicle is level with the floor of the warehouse. Dock-leveling devices are available to suit vehicles of different heights.

4. Plan the medical store with staging areas for preparing shipments (issuing) and unloading deliveries (receiving). Separate the receiving and shipping areas to avoid confusion and to enhance efficiency and security. Other operation areas required in most warehouses are reserve storage, picking, packing, returns, and value added services.

Store aisle layout principles

Picking face towards the assembly area
where very frequent access is required

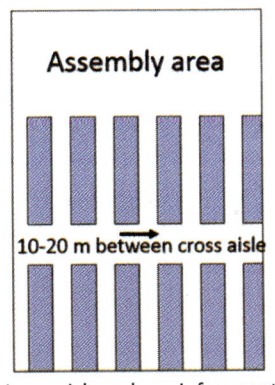

Long aisles where infrequent access is required

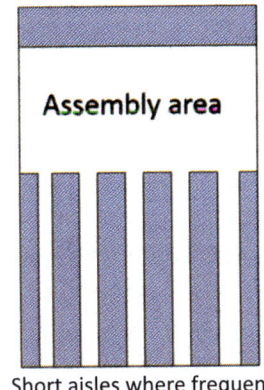

Short aisles where frequent access is required

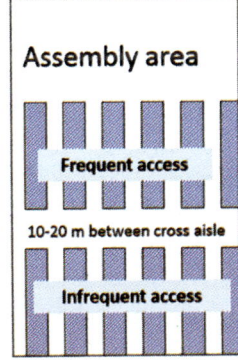

Combined arrangement

5. If a facility will be repackaging products, plan a separate clean preparation area to conduct the repackaging. Try to locate the area close to the issuing area.

6. **Cold storage:** In larger facilities it is more efficient to use cold rooms rather than numerous refrigerators or freezers (which generate heat). Ideally, larger facilities should have one room with a negative temperature for frozen products (-20°C) and another room with a positive but cold temperature (2°-8°C) for products requiring refrigeration.

7. **Secure storage:** All medical stores should have a secure storage are for products that are likely to be stolen or abused. A locked cabinet or cupboard may be sufficient for some facilities, while other facilities may require a vault or cage.

8. **Ventilation:** The location and design should ensure maximum air circulation to avoid concentrations of fumes or gases and to prevent condensation of moisture on products or walls. Use an extractor fan to remove fumes, gases, and moisture.

9. **Fire precautions:** Certain pharmaceuticals, flammables, hazardous drugs and dangerous materials should be located in separate store independent of the main building or in a fire-proof compartment within it. Fire protection must be to a standard at least as high as required by the local building codes for hazardous chemical stores. If contained within the main warehouse, one wall should be external and should contain large ventilator grills positioned so as to enable a fire to vent outwards without risk to the main structure or to the surrounding buildings,

   All sections of the warehouse should have adequate fire detection equipment and be well supplied with the fire -fighting appliances.

10. **Roof and ceiling:** Design a slanting roof to allow water run-off. Extend the roof over the windows to give extra protection from rain and direct sunlight.

    Install a double ceiling to provide insulation and ensure that supplies are kept cool.

11. **Walls and floor:** The walls and floors of a medical store should be permanent and smooth for easy cleaning. Walls preferably should be constructed of brick or concrete blocks. Perforated or bored bricks might be used for the upper portion of the wall to allow ventilation, but these should be screened to prevent the entry of rodents and other pests. Construct or treat floors of larger facilities to ensure they can withstand the frequent movement of heavy products and equipment. This should be done with the guidance of an engineer. The floor must be able to carry product loads, as well as support rack post and forklift equipment, without causing short- and long-term damage to the floor.

12. **Doors:** Plan doors wide enough to allow for the free and easy movement of supplies and handling equipment. Large facilities, such as those at the central level, often use forklifts and other handling equipment. Ensure doors are strong and reinforced to provide adequate security. Fit them with two strong locks, and install metal grills for extra protection.

13. **Lighting:** Plan the storeroom with as much natural light (sunlight) in the day as possible to avoid the use of either fluorescent or incandescent bulb lighting. Fluorescent lighting emits ultraviolet rays, which have a negative effect on certain products. Incandescent bulbs emit heat. At the same time, take care to ensure that products are not in direct sunlight.

    Adequate electrical lighting is required throughout the store.

14. **Windows:** Plan windows that are high and wide to allow adequate ventilation. They should be high enough to not be blocked by shelves, have wire mesh to keep out insect, and be burglar proofed.

15. **Cupboards:** Provide cupboards for the storage of specific products that must be kept free from dust or light.

16. **Shelves:** The exact position of racking and shelving should be developed to ensure that everything will fit when implemented. The layout design has a significant influence on order-picking and travelling distances in the warehouse. Computer Aided Designs (CAD) programme and process or similar technology can be utilized, if available to design detailed warehouse

layout. CAD can help generate multiple variations of layouts for departments, flow, rack positions, conveyor, sortation and material handling. Arrange shelves and racks in lines with a passageway not less than 90 cm wide. Avoid placing shelves only around the edge of the room, which wastes a lot of space. Place the shelves 90 cm from the walls of the storeroom to ensure they are accessible from both sides. Ideally, use adjustable shelves.

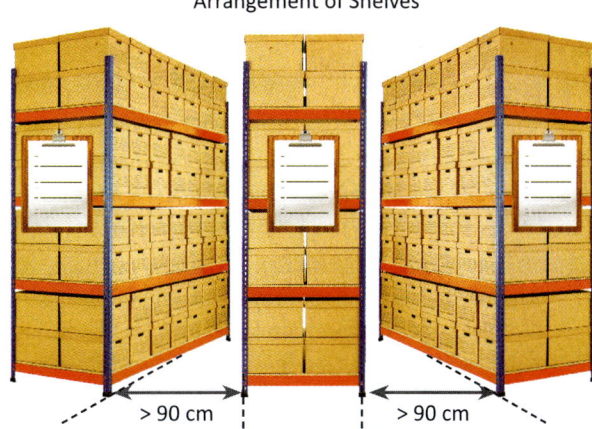

Arrangement of Shelves

> 90 cm   > 90 cm

III. MATERIALS HANDLING EQUIPMENT AND STORAGE MEDIA

Match storage modes, IT systems, radio frequency identification devices (RFID) and mechanized technologies with volumes. Equipments include static racking equipment, mezzanines or alike, or mechanical equipment such as conveyors, horizontal/vertical carousels (a conveyor system manual or for automated picking), stacker cranes, etc. must be applied according to their purpose, limitations and suitability for the volumes to be handled. Follow simple rule to keep manual handling of products to a minimum; ideally no more than 3-5 touches while goods are in the warehouse.

1. **Shelves and cupboards:** Use shelves and cupboards to store smaller products. Adjust the shelves as needed to allow for packages of different sizes.

2. **Tables in the packing area:** Provide large tables in the packing area for staff to use when assembling and packing shipments. Keep the tables clean.

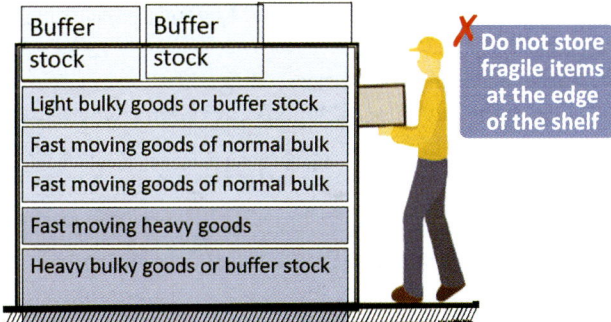

Shelf layout for variable picking frequencies

Buffer stock	Buffer stock	
Light bulky goods or buffer stock		
Fast moving goods of normal bulk		
Fast moving goods of normal bulk		
Fast moving heavy goods		
Heavy bulky goods or buffer stock		

✗ Do not store fragile items at the edge of the shelf

3. **Pallets:** Pallets are used to store bulk items and larger cartons. They keep things off the floor and can be used with forklifts or trolleys to move around groups of larger items. Pallets are generally used only in larger facilities because storing and moving pallets can be expensive. Smaller facilities might may make their own shelves using planks of wood supported on bricks or crates, if there is no shelving in the storeroom to keep products off the shore.

4. If facility uses pallets, remember to:

   i. Always inspect pallets before loading them with material. Ensure that pallets are solid and sturdy with no loose or cracked boards and no protruding nails. Damaged pallets can break while being lifted and cause serious injuries and product damage.

   ii. Pile empty pallets neatly and out of aisles.

iii. If possible, keep pallets indoors, away from elements that can gradually break down the wood.

iv. Do NOT mix different types of products on one pallet.

v. Do NOT mix different batches of the same product on one pallet.

5. Regardless of the material they are made of, pallets increase the risk of fire because they provide open space for oxygen to fuel a fire and a large surface area for a fire to burn. Always follow the safety precautions discussed in the fire protection section of this book.

6. Shelves, cupboards, tables, and pallets can be made of wood, metal, and plastic. Metal shelves, cupboards, and pallets may be steel, stainless steel, or aluminum. These tend to cost more, but are stronger, more durable, and less flammable than plastic or wood. Also they are not vulnerable to insect, rodent, or fungus problems.

Storage and handling equipment

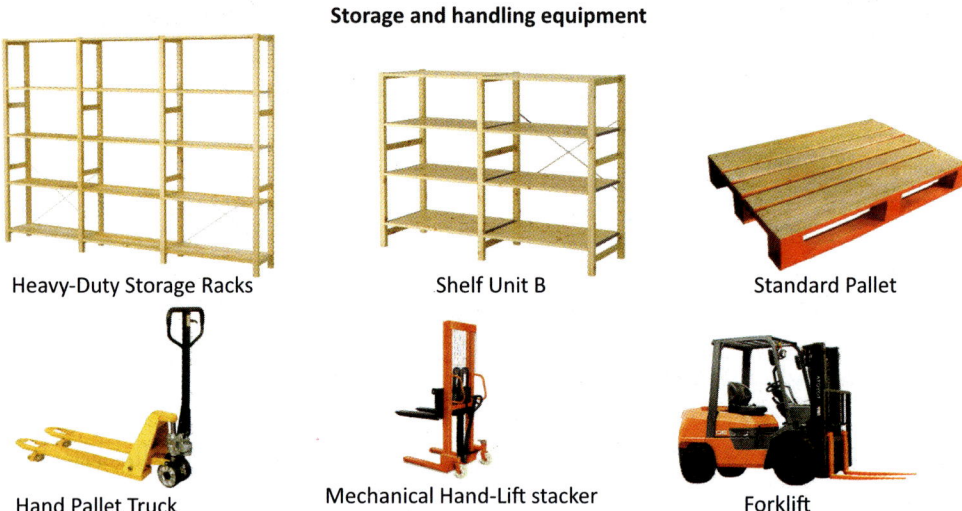

Heavy-Duty Storage Racks   Shelf Unit B   Standard Pallet

Hand Pallet Truck   Mechanical Hand-Lift stacker   Forklift

7. Forklifts and pallet lifters: Pallet lifters come in two types, walkie and seated, and each has some advantages. Walkies are better when space is limited because the turning radius is smaller. However, they are very slow moving and are not as useful in larger warehouses. Seated lifters move much faster but are much more expensive.

8. If plan is to use forklifts or pallet lifters in the facility:

i. Ensure the floor is even and able to withstand the weight of the loaded lifter.

ii. Ensure the lifter has room to load and unload products.

iii. Consider the appropriate lifter for your facility. Forklifts and pallet lifters can be powered by gas, diesel, liquid propane gas, or electricity, all of which affect the capacity and cost. Also consider the warehouse ventilation and environment.

iv. Keep an extra battery or a battery charger, if needed. Ensure the battery can last a full day.

v. Ensure the lifter can reach the highest pallet rack.

vi. Keep a record of maintenance and servicing of the lifter in a secure, visible place.

vii. Maintain and post picture identification of employees who have been trained and are authorized to operate the lifter.

15 | Quality Tools in Pharmacy and Medical Stores

Low-resource pharmacies face unique efficiency challenges such as manpower and space. The pharmacist's major responsibility is to spend more time on tasks which add value, such as education and counselling of patients on how to take medicines. On the contrary pharmacists spend the majority of their time on non–value-added tasks leading to waste. The pharmacy department can benefit significantly from applying quality tools and techniques to its inpatient pharmacy. Quality tools are used for quality improvement informed by both Lean and Six Sigma practices.

A. INTRODUCTION TO QUALITY

Lean and Six Sigma were developed separately in the automotive and telecommunications industries, respectively, to increase efficiency and quality. The foundation of Lean processing began with the Toyota family in Japan in the early 1900s. The philosophy of Lean is reduction of waste in order to improve production and reduce cost. Six Sigma was designed to reduce cost by decreasing defects. Defects are one of the most visible examples of waste and can be easy to grasp in any sector or industry. Six Sigma was first developed by Motorola in 1986 and made popular in the mid-1990s by General Electric.

Defects refer to any product or service that doesn't meet commercial specifications and must be discarded, or fixed via additional resources. Defects can cause waste in numerous ways in addition to the capital used to scrap or rebuild a product or service. Defects affect delivery times, logistics, and ultimately customer satisfaction. It is desirable not to spend an extra second on the rescheduling, paperwork and critical thinking that goes into fixing defects. Excess inventory, is an example of overproduction which then leads to additional expenditure on storage space and preservation. This does not add value. Long waiting to be served at the pharmacy results in dissatisfied patients. Transportation waste involves the unnecessary movement of product or information that doesn't add value. This comes in the form of moving a process from one individual to another, within the same department, and to another department. All of this adds unnecessary time onto a process. To eliminate this kind of waste, one can combine tasks and roles, and in extreme cases, reorganize workspaces to reduce physical movement (see below).

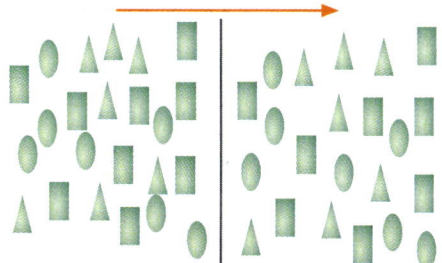

Searching for a missing item - time spent 10 minutes

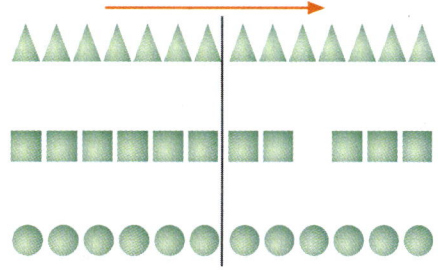

Searching for a missing item - With Sort & Set time spent 2 seconds

Reorganize workspaces to reduce time in tracing the items.

Motion is any process that takes up time or capital by employees or machines, that fails to add value to the activity. Making duplicate repetitious entries in registers which does not add any value in monitoring or performance is another waste.

Common reasons for waste include:

- Poor process design and controls
- Poor workstation/store layout
- Shared tools and machines
- Workstation congestion
- Isolated and siloed operations
- Lack of standard

The combination of both techniques (Lean and Six Sigma) for the purpose of quality improvement is termed Lean Six Sigma (LSS). While both techniques began in manufacturing years ago, their adoption into health care has increased recently only as institutions have found themselves pressed to increase quality while simultaneously decreasing costs.

LSS principles allow pharmacies to drastically improve processes to improve quality for customers. A department does not need a great deal of resources or expertise to implement LSS principles and reap the rewards. Creative use of willing volunteers can produce results quickly.

B. LEAN SIX SIGMA (LSS) TERMINOLOGY

Lean Six Sigma Terminology

Lean Six Sigma Terminology	Description
Lean	A practice to maximize value, as defined by the customer, and minimizes waste.
Value added	Anything for which a customer would pay.
Non-value added	Any activity that does not contribute to adding customer-defined value.
Gemba walk	Gemba is a Japanese term for where the work occurs. A gemba walk is going to where the work occurs in order to learn granular information about the work process. For example, where do the delays occur? What is the current process? Where do defects occur?
Kanban	Kanban cards describe when to order an item, how much to order, and the item's order number were created (see below).
Value stream mapping (VSM)	Analyzing the current work flow and identifying waste, focusing on areas of bottlenecks and decreased efficiency.
Lean Six Sigma (LSS) events	Various names are applied to describe different types of events. LSS events range from short 1-half or 1-day events (Express Workout), to 3- to 5-day.
Kaizen	LSS events, called kaizens. Kaizen is the Japanese word meaning "improvement." Kaizen or continuous improvement is about doing "little things" better everyday. It is slow, gradual but continuous improvement. Problem solving under Kaizen is a cross functional, systematic and collaborative approach.
5S Principles	Sort, set in order, shine, standardize, and systemize.

Sample Kanban card containing prescriptive descriptions on how to complete a process or part of a process.

KANBAN CARD

Item Name: Paracetamol

Item number: XYZ

Supplier name: ABC

Reorder quantity: 2 boxes (100 packs)

Procedure

1. **Request order:** to place it in items 'to order bin' when you see Kanban

2. **Place order:** once order is placed put Kanban in 'Awaiting delivery bin'

3. **Receive delivery:** Once item is delivered, check 'Awaiting delivery' bin for the matching Kanban

4. **Return Kanban:** Stock item at a correct location using FEFO; place new item behind existing inventory

---

C. 5S IN PHARMACY

1. 5S is a lean method for workplace organization; it represents a way of focusing and thinking in order to better organize and manage workspace, specifically by eliminating the wastes.

2. The application of 5S helps organize the workplace starting from physical environment and gradually to functional aspects. The application of 5S simplifies the activities through reduction of waste and unproductive/unnecessary activities. It is also helpful in improving the quality, efficiency and safety.

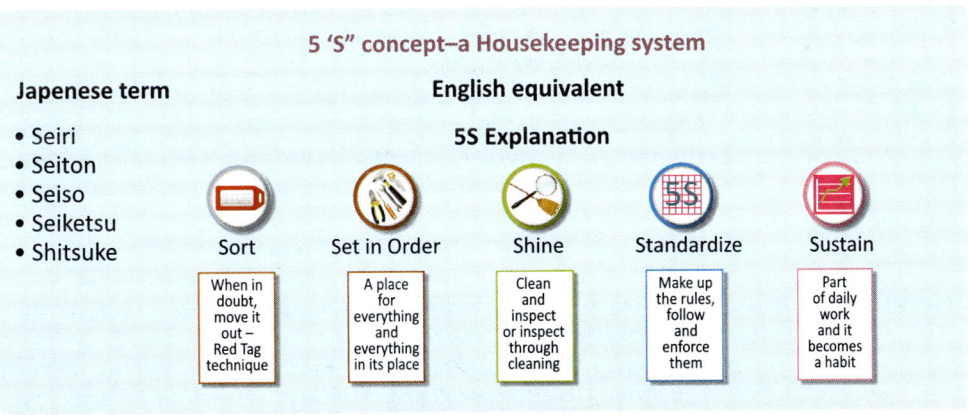

5 'S" concept–a Housekeeping system

Japenese term	English equivalent				
• Seiri	**5S Explanation**				
• Seiton					
• Seiso	Sort	Set in Order	Shine	Standardize	Sustain
• Seiketsu					
• Shitsuke	When in doubt, move it out – Red Tag technique	A place for everything and everything in its place	Clean and inspect or inspect through cleaning	Make up the rules, follow and enforce them	Part of daily work and it becomes a habit

3. The 5S management method is recognized as the foundation of lean healthcare approaches, which maximize value-added levels by removing all factors that do not generate values. Also, the concept of "a place for everything and everything in its place," is the backbone of 5S. It allows for ease in identification of waste and non-conformance when the workplace is not in proper order. This focus on the identification and elimination of waste is, the most basic tenet of Lean and, while most organizations clearly understand the need for and practice excellence in keeping the workplace "clean," they are often very poor at keeping that same workplace "organized" and "orderly." 5S examples in pharmacy are shown in Table below:

5S in pharmacy and examples

Japanese	English	Actions/Examples
Seiri	Sort	Identify and remove unwanted/unused items from the workplace; and reduce clutter (Removal/organization)
		• Waste disposal, both infectious and non-infectious
		• Timely condemnation of unwanted stores and a separate condemn items stores.
		• Initiation of "Reduce, Reuse, Recycle Concept"; Items, which can be provided to the safe recycling process, for instance, inner wrapping paper of disposable surgical gloves, glass bottles of IV antibiotics/equipment and so forth.
		• Benefits include: a more effective use of space, simplified tasks, a reduction in hazards, and a significant decrease in distracting clutter.
Seiton	Set in Order	"Set" based on perfection of "Sort".
		Organize everything needed in proper order for easy operation (Orderliness). With an organized and efficient use of storage, everyone is easily able to locate important items and enjoy a less stressful work environment. Examples include:
		• Items are arranged according to alphabetical order or numerical order. All the items should be kept in a specific place following a system, so that anybody in need of these items can find them easily.
		• Name tag, board and symbols development and installation. Identify names of all the rooms and install a simple board for easy recognition by the staff and visitors.
		• Digital token, separate queue at pharmacy counter and separate waiting space at OPD and pharmacy to avoid confusion, congestion and conflict.
		• To classify patients and visitors coming to the hospital (as patients with urgent attendance, on the first visit, and the patients seeking re-examination).
		• Tagging and labelling of all the items, instruments and devices
		• Specific locations for the items, arranging workable instrument sets, storage of these sets, and colour coding system for easy handling.
Seiso	Shine	Maintain high standard of cleanliness (Cleanness). Employees will feel more comfortable in this clean and uncluttered environment
		• Checklist of cleaning activities
		• Daily 10 minutes morning "Shine" practice before starting routine work.
		• Achieve Shine by cleaning tools - cleaning tool renewal, assigning tool storage, space arrangement and provision of small office and better uniform for cleaning staff.
		• "Shine" should be applied at waste separation, collection, storage, transport and final treatment system
		• Prevent entry of insects, animals (especially rodents) or birds
		• Walls must be finished in a smooth, impervious, washable material
Seiketsu	Standardize	Set up the above 5S as norms in every section of the workplace (Standardize)
		• Pre-packaging of frequently used drug.
		• Labelling: Arranging the necessary items at the appropriate place with proper numbering, labelling and colour code makes it easy to find out quickly.
		• Uniform colour code system. e.g., "blue" to indicate sterile materials, while "red" is used for unsterile items.
		• Regular supervisory visits
		• Informal site visits to supervise the ongoing 5S activities
Shitsuke	Sustain	Train and maintain discipline of the personnel engaged (Self-Discipline) - Short (usually one topic) but practical training
		• Create positive competition
		• Safety issues and 5S activities
		• Effective hospital accident or incident (to hospital staff, visitors or patients) reporting system

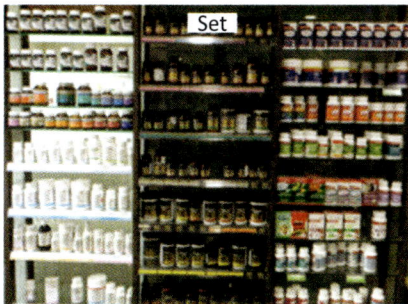

All items set in their place

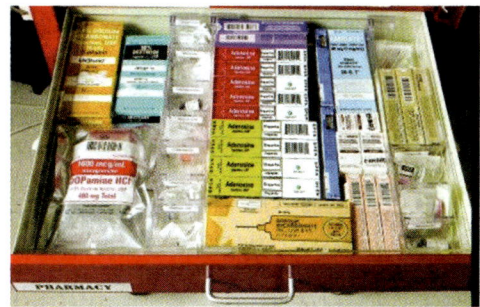

Drawer also a sort and set target

Sort and Set by organizing everything needed in proper order for easy operation (Orderliness) such as arranging stores alphabetically or dosage forms

D. USING LSS IN PHARMACY

Steps for using LSS in pharmacy

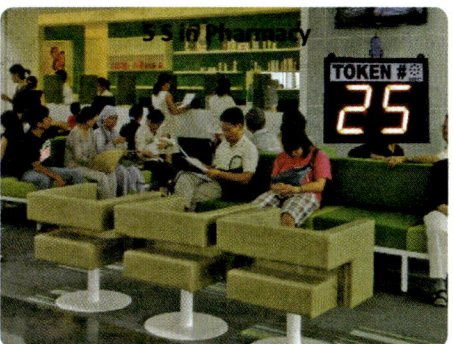

Digital token, separate queue at ticket counter and separate waiting space at Pharmacy

1.   Identify the problem you want to solve or process you want to improve

2.   Gain support from management and individuals willing to join the team

3.   Create a team

4.   Become intimately knowledgeable about the current work process

5.   Conduct a gemba walk (an observation of the work process)

6.   Understand the value stream

7.   Keep the customers in the forefront

8.   Choose solutions based on predicted high impact (see below)

9.   Implement changes

10. Ensure that there are measures for accountability

11. Promote continued quality improvement i.e., standardization of the improvements, and routine monitoring and tracking of improvements following implementation.

12. Credit performance of team members.

LSS projects can be utilized on a small or large scale. The first important task is to identify a process that needs to be improved. Gather the proper support to conduct an LSS event. If the pharmacy group is small, invite colleagues from other disciplines to help. Allowing staff to be creative in forming teams can yield great results. Interdisciplinary members' perspectives contribute fresh and valuable ideas. It is important to have support from management whether in the form of their participation or support to help eliminate obstacles that might be hindering the identified process. Create a team based on the anticipated workload of the project. If the project is larger than your volunteer pool, limit the scope of the project to a smaller piece of the overall problem.

After the team is formed, every team member should understand the current work process. The gemba walk is a way to ensure that all members observe the work flow. The next step is to prepare for a Kaizen improvement activity. Kaizen is a Japanese word that means change for the better, or more commonly, continuous improvement. A Kaizen is a hands-on burst of improvement activity in the actual workspace that occurs during a relatively short period of time – usually three or four days. Brain storm improvement approaches with a team, which was comprised of those who perform the activities everyday. Once the team feels comfortable with the process, brainstorm potential improvements that could improve value for the customer. Then test them (called "trystorming") on the actual production or service line. To determine what the value for the customer is, the customers must be identified. Although patients are an obvious end point, nurses and others who rely on pharmacy must be kept in the forefront of improvement efforts. Delivering value to the customer should be the focus. Speaking with customers or creating surveys, prior to the LSS event, are helpful ways to gather data regarding customer value.

Next step is brainstorm potential solutions. This method results in rapid recognition of which solutions will work and which will not. The Kaizen team also creates plans to sustain the gains once improvements were made, and developed reports to leadership on its actions. The team can create criteria for determining what constitutes high and low effort and impact. Remain consistent throughout the ranking process. The goal is to identify processes that can be improved with little effort, but that will yield high impact. Proceed with solutions that are deemed to be high impact and low effort. Although this is a good way to identify starting points, the team may be flexible in pursuing high-effort projects that must be completed or low-impact but easily completed projects.

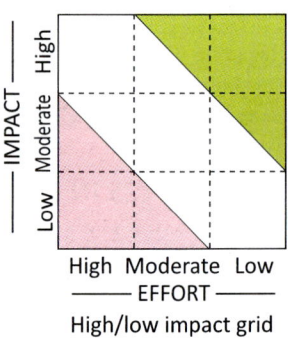

High/low impact grid

E. EXAMPLE OF QUALITY IMPROVEMENT INITIATIVES

In a pharmacy facing physical space constraints— The immediate solutions appear to expand with more space. However, undertaking initial activity centred on a 5S of the pharmacy (sort, set in order, shine, standardize and sustain) can free up lot of space. These 5S activities can include evaluation of the purpose and value of all supplies and activities in the work areas. This step alone

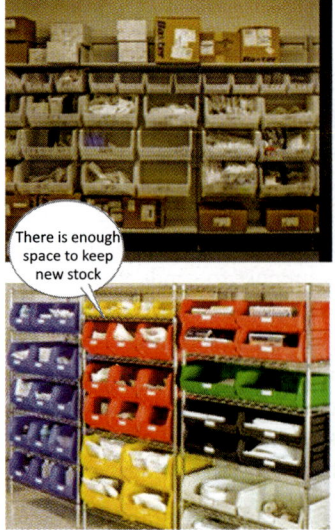
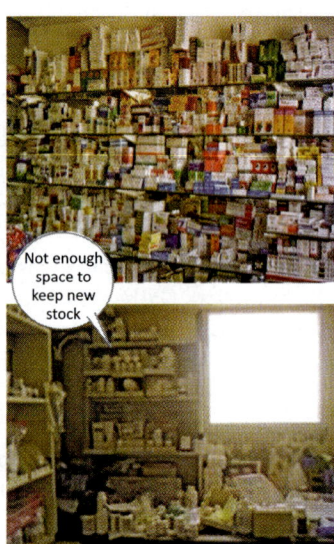

Using 5S to decide options (to dejunk or expand) to a
pharmacy facing physical storage space constraint.

clears a significant amount of "clutter" from the area, improving visual control and eliminating several safety hazards. The 5S activity can free up an entire rack where medication that was no longer used was being stored. (such as expired drugs, empty cartons, old records).

Second step would be to set up a "Unwanted Items Store" or "Condemning Store". This store is used to collect unwanted items from all work units or departments after commencing "Sort" step of 5S. Each unit actively removes unwanted, unnecessary, unworkable items from their venues and brings them to the store. Since those items are all government property, the hospital cannot discard them immediately. Due to this nature, the items have to be kept for a while until the permission is granted by the authority. At the store, the items should be further classified into several subgroups. Functioning, broken but reparable, irreparable, and clutter are the subcategories.

FURTHER READING

1. Drugs & Cosmetics Act, 1940 and the Drugs & Cosmetics Rules, 1945. Akalank Publications, 1995.

2. Drugs & Therapeutic Committees: A Practical Guide. World Health Organization in Collaboration with Management Sciences for Health. WHO/EDM/PAR/2004.1.

3. Good Pharmacy Practice Guidelines. Guidelines for delivery of Pharmaceutical Services and care in Community Pharmacy Settings in India. Community Pharmacy Division. Indian Pharmaceutical Association, India. March 2002.

4. Good Pharmacy Practice in South Africa. The South African Pharmacy Council. December 2003.

5. Good Storage Practices for Pharmaceutical Products at a Retail Pharmacy: A Guide for Retail Pharmacists/dispensers. Delhi Pharmaceutical Trust, New Delhi.

6. Guidelines for Storage of Essential Drugs and other Health Commodities. DELIVER in collaboration with the World Health Organization and UNICEF.

7. Managing Drug Supply. Management Sciences for Health in collaboration with World Health Organization. Quick JD, Rankin JR, Laing RO, O'Connor RW, Hogerzeil HV, Dukes MNG and Garnett A (eds). Second edition, Kumarian Press 1997.

8. Operational Principles for Good Pharmaceutical Procurement. World Health Organization, Geneva. WHO/EDM/PAR/99.5.

9. Practical Guidelines on Pharmaceutical Procurement for Countries with small Procurement Agencies. World Health Organization, Regional office for the Western Pacific, Manila, Philippines 2002.

10. IAP Guide Book on Immunization. Committee on Immunization. Indian Academy of Paediatrics.

11. Cold chain: management for vaccine handler. Minsitry of Health & Family Welfare, Nirman Bhawan, New Delhi.

12. Practical guidelines on pharmaceutical procurement for countries with small procurement agencies. World Health Organization, Regional office for the Western Pacific, Manila, Philippines 2002.

13. https://www.who.int/medicines/areas/quality_safety/quality_assurance/ GoodDistributionPracticesTRS957Annex5.pdf

14. EADSG Guidelines: Insulin Storage and Optimisation of Injection Technique in Diabetes Management. Diabetes Ther. 2019 Apr; 10(2): 341–366. doi: HYPERLINK "https://dx.doi.org/10.1007%2Fs13300-019-0574-x"10.1007/s13300-019-0574-x

APPENDIX 1a: Key Indian Regulations & Guidelines

Regulation/Guideline	Description
Central Drugs Standard Control Organization (CDSCO)	Ministry of Health & Family Welfare, Government of India provides general information about drug regulatory requirements in India.
National Pharmaceutical Pricing Authority (NPPA)	Drugs (Price Control) Order 1995 and other orders enforced by Government of India. View the list of drugs under price control.
Drugs & Cosmetic (D & C) Act, 1940	The Drugs & Cosmetics Act, 1940 regulates the import, manufacture, distribution and sale of drugs in India.
Good Clinical Practice (GCP) guidelines	The Ministry of Health, along with Drugs Controller General of India (DCGI) and Indian Council for Medical Research (ICMR) has come out with guidelines for research in human subjects. These GCP guidelines are essentially based on Declaration of Helsinki, WHO guidelines and ICH requirements for good clinical practice.
The Pharmacy Act, 1948	The Pharmacy Act, 1948 is meant to regulate the profession of Pharmacy in India.
The Drugs and Magic Remedies (Objectionable Advertisement) Act, 1954	The Drugs and Magic Remedies (Objectionable Advertisement) Act, 1954 provides to control the advertisements regarding drugs; it prohibits the advertising of remedies alleged to possess magic qualities.
The Narcotic Drugs and Psychotropic Substances (NDPS) Act, 1985	NDPS is an act concerned with control and regulation of operations relating to Narcotic Drugs and Psychotropic Substances.
Pharmacy Practice Rules And Regulations 2015	Pharmacy Practice Rules 2015 seek to address the rights of pharmacists. These regulation allow concept of Pharma clinic and finally gives pharmacists their rightful role in healthcare.

APPENDIX 1b: Drugs and Cosmetic Act, 1940 Schedules

Schedule	Description
Schedule G	Details of drugs to be labeled with words "Caution – it is dangerous to take this preparation except under medical supervision e.g. insulin, metformin, promethazine, etc.
Schedule H	Deals with drugs and medicines, which must be sold by retail only when a prescription by registered medical practitioner is produced e.g. Captopril, atenolol, allopurinol, haloperidol, norfloxacin, etc.
Schedule H1	Deals with a class of prescription drugs which should be sold on prescription of a registered practitioner and record of the same to be maintained by the dispensing pharmacist. It includes 47 medicines (3rd and 4th generation antibiotics, antitubercular drugs and certain habit forming drugs like psychotropic drugs). The schedule H1 drugs should be labeled with the symbol Rx in red, clearly displayed on the left top corner of the drug label. The label should also bear the following words in the box with a red border: Schedule H1 drug – warning • It is dangerous to take this preparation except in accordance with the medical advice • Not to be sold by retail without the prescription of a registered medical practitioner At the time of dispensing record should be maintained in a register mentioning about the name and address of the prescriber, name of the patient and name of the drug alongwith quantity supplied. The register should be kept for three years and should be open for inspection.
Schedule K	Consists of drugs supplied by a registered medical practitioner to his own patient exempted from the provisions of Chapter IV of the Act and the Rules. All the provisions of Chapter IV of the Act and the Rules are subject to the following conditions: The drugs shall be purchased only from a dealer or a manufacturer licensed under these rules and records of such purchases to be maintained. In the case of medicine containing a substance specified in Schedule G, H or X the additional conditions as required should be complied with. It includes household remedies like aspirin tab, paracetamol tab, analgesic balm, gripe water for use of infants, etc.; Substances which are used both as articles of food as well as drugs; Drugs supplied by hospital or supported by government or local body.
Schedule J	Disease and ailment (by whatever name described), which a drug may not purport to prevent or cure e.g. Appendicitis, blindness, blood poisoning, blood pressure (high or low), etc.
Schedule M	Specifies the general and specific requirements for factory premises and materials, plant and equipment and minimum recommended areas for basic installation for certain categories of drugs.
Schedule N	Deals with minimum equipments of a pharmacy and gives direction regarding (a) entrance of a pharmacy (b) premises (c) furniture and apparatus (d) general provisions.
Schedule P	Defines life period of drugs (shelf life), the period up to which the drug will remain stable under the storage conditions from the date of manufacture.
Schedule W	List of drugs that shall be marketed under generic name only.
Schedule X	Gives the name of psychotropic drugs, requiring special license for manufacture and sale e.g. Morphine, amfepramone, barbital, benzphetamine, etc.
Schedule Y	Specifications for the clinical trials legislative requirements.

APPENDIX 1C: DEFINITION OF SUBSTANDARD DRUGS

MISBRANDED DRUGS

A drug shall be deemed to be misbranded:

a.   If it is so coloured, coated, powered or polished that damage is concealed or if it is made to appear of better or greater therapeutic value than it really is; or

b.   If it is not labeled in the prescribed manner; or

c.   If it is label or container or anything accompanying the drug bears any statement design or device, which makes any false claim for, the drug.

ADULTERATED DRUGS

A drug shall be deemed to be adulterated:

a.   If it consists in whole or in part, of any filthy, putrified or decomposed substance, or

b.   If it has been prepared, packed or stored under unsanitary conditions whereby it may have been contaminated with filth or whereby it may have been rendered injurious to health or

c.   If as container is composed, in whole or in part of any poisonous or deleterious substance which may render the contents injurious to health; or

d.   If it bears or contains, for purposes of colouring only, a colour other than one which is prescribed, or

e.   If any substance has been mixed therewith so as to reduce its quality or strength.

SPURIOUS DRUGS

A drug shall be deemed to be spurious:

a.   If it is manufactured under a name which belongs to another drug; or

b.   If it is an imitation of or is a substitute for, another drug or resembles another drug in a manner likely to deceive or bears upon it or upon its label or container the name of another drug unless it is plainly and conspicuously marked so as to reveal its true character and its lack of identity with such other drug; or

c.   If the label container bears the name of an individual or company purporting to be the manufacturer of the drug, which individual or company is fictitious or does not exist; or

d.   If it has been substituted wholly or in part by another drug or substance; or

e.   If it purports to be the product of a manufacturer of whom it is not truly a product.

APPENDIX 2: Discrepancy Report

DISCREPANCY REPORT

Health facility: Charama CHC

Date : 18.04.2014

1. Received by: Narender Mohan

No. of cartons received: 03

2. Witnessed by: Deepak

No. of other containers received: 01

DETAILS OF SHIPMENT

3. Issue voucher no.: 98570

Vehicle reg. no.: CH 1532

4. Transporter: DHS Driver

Transporter shipment note:

5. Name of driver: Mahender

List of cartons not received: 1 container 5 liter

6. List of cartons received.: 03

_____

DETAILS OF DISCREPANCIES

7. Breakages (if any):

Issue voucher no.	Item Description	Code No.	Unit	Quantity Broken
98570	Chloroquine syrup	03-2500	Bottle 500ml	2

8. Items missing:

Issue voucher no.	Item Description	Code No..	Unit	Quantity Missing
98570	Chlorhexidine solution 2%	04-1650	5 liter	1

9. Items issued in error:

Issue voucher no.	Item Description	Code No.	Unit	Quantity Tampered with

10. Any other discrepancies /comments:

Please credit breakages and resupply any missing items

11. Signature: Office held:

APPENDIX 3: Receiving Report

RECEIVING REPORT

Supplier: Apotex Inc.

PO No.: DMS – 116/17

Port of entry: Port S. Philip

Date received at port of entry: 05/12/98

Number of shipping cartons/containers: 3

Invoice No.: 686033

Carrier: Fast Forwarders

Date Cleared: 05/17/18

Certified that from external inspections, all containers appear to be suitable and without damage except as follows:

_____

_____

_____

Clearing Officer   Date:

Certified that all items on the invoice and the purchase order (specified above) were received and after inspection, released for removal to shelving except as follows (or as marked on the invoice).

Receiving clerk   Date: Chief storekeeper   Date:

APPENDIX 4: Sample Register

Description: Paracetamol tabs 500 mg   Unit of issue: 1000 tabs

Stock No.: 02-

UNIT		MAXIMUM STOCK		MINIMUM STOCK		LOCATION		
Date 2019	Document/ Number	Received From/ Issued to	Units received	Units issued	Losses / Adjustments	Balance	Qty on order	Initials
Mar 5		Balance Brought Forward						
Mar 5	N 98534	PHC 42		10		1655		RS
Mar 6	N98543	HOSP 6		200		1445		RS
Mar 6	N98546	PHC 55		16		1429		BJ
Mar 6	N98561	PHC 53		10		1419		PF
Mar 7	N98573	PHC 66		5		1232		RS
Mar 7	N98575	PHC 62		5		1227		RS
Mar 7	N98574	PHC 68		5		1212		RS
Mar 8	N98166	NOVAPHARM	10000			11202		BJ
Mar 8	N98605	HOSP 9		200		11002		BJ
Mar 8	N98604	HOSP 8		200		10802		BJ
Mar 8	N98609	PHC71		10		10729		RS
Mar 8	N98613	PHC 78		12		10770		RS

APPENDIX 5: Sample Requisition/Issue Voucher

Requisition no.: _____

Health Facility: _____

Authorized by: _____

Date: _____   Supply period _____ to _____

Item No.	Stock Number	Description	Unit of Issue	Stock on Hand	Quantity Requested	Quantity Approved	Quantity Issued	Amount (Rs.)	Notes
1	2	2	3	4	5	6	7	8	9
1	02-0500	Aspirin tabs 300mg	1000T	12	18	18	18	165.60	
2	02-2200	Chloroquine tabs 150mg	1000T	3	5	5	5	61.00	
18	02-4600	Paracetamol tabs 500mg	1000T	6	8	8	8	209.60	
19	02-4800	Phenoxymethyl tabs 250mg	1000T	3	4	4	2	81.40	Short
20	02-4850	Piperazine tabs 500mg	1000T	1	1	1	1	11.20	

Hour and date requisition received _____   Hour and date consignment received _____

CLEARANCES:

1. Shipping and receiving review   2. In-charge of medical stores   3. Inventory control unit

4. Medical stores   5. Shipping and receiving   6. Driver or custodian accepts shipment

7. Recipient, acknowledgment of receipt of shipment

APPENDIX 6: Sample Bin/Stock Card

Description: Paracetamol tabs 500 mg **Unit of issue: 1000 tabs**

Stock No.: 02-

UNIT		MAXIMUM STOCK	MINIMUM STOCK	LOCATION		
Date 2018		Units received	Unites issued	Balance	Initials	
Mar 5						
Mar 5			10	1655	RS	
Mar 6			200	1445	RS	
Mar 6			16	1429	BJ	
Mar 6			10	1419	PF	
Mar 7			5	1232	RS	
Mar 7			5	1227	RS	
Mar 7			5	1212	RS	
Mar 8		10000		11202	BJ	
Mar 8			200	11002	BJ	
Mar 8			200	10802	BJ	
Mar 8			10	10729	RS	
Mar 8			12	10770	RS	

APPENDIX 7: Delivery Voucher

Deliver to: _____

Requisition No.: _____   Issue voucher No.: _____

Received from Central/District Medical Stores _____ sealed cartons and containers described below:

for delivery to the above- named requisitioner/facility

_____   _____

Stores issuing officer   Driver/custodian of shipment   Date and time

Received by requisitioner from the above-named custodian of shipment, the containers and/or items stated above in good order, except as follows:

_____   _____

Receiving officer of requisitioning facility   Date and time

IF ANY DISCREPANCY IS RECORDED BY THE RECEIVING OFFICER, THIS DELIVERY VOUCHER IS TO BE INITIALED BY THE CUSTODIAN OF THE SHIPMENT AS WELL

APPENDIX 8: Sample Register of Requisitions

(STORES ISSUES LEDGER)

Stores Issue No.	Date	Requisition No.	Issue Voucher No.	Drugs	Med. Surg.	Other	Total	Certified
					Value of Issues (Rs.)			
001	Mar 5	98-3-2R	PHC 42 98534	2412.60	836.50	---	3249.10	Ramnarayan
002	Mar 5	98-3-2R	PHC44 98541	2933.50	1078.50	---	4012.00	Ramnarayan
003	Mar 5	98-3-4R	HOSP6 98543-45	28364.20	6517.60	937.50	35819.30	Ramnarayan
023	Mar 8	98-3-4R	PHC75 98611	3545.30	948.60	---	4493.90	Madhav
024	Mar 8	98-3-4R	PHC78 98613	2266.40	592.30	---	2858.70	Madhav
025	Mar 8	98-3-4R	PHC72 98614	2947.70	876.10	---	3823.80	Madhav

Index